Death, Dying, and Social Differences

Death, Dying, and Social Differences

SECOND EDITION

Edited by

David Oliviere
Director of Education and Training,
St Christopher's Hospice, Sydenham, London, UK
Visiting Professor, Middlesex University, London, UK

Barbara Monroe
Chief Executive, St Christopher's Hospice,
Sydenham, London, UK
Honorary Professor, International Observatory on End of
Life Care, Lancaster University, Lancaster, UK

Sheila Payne
Director of the International Observatory on End of Life Care,
and Help the Hospices Chair in Hospice Studies,
Lancaster University, Lancaster, UK
Director of the Cancer Experiences Collaborative, UK

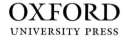
OXFORD
UNIVERSITY PRESS

OXFORD

UNIVERSITY PRESS

Great Clarendon Street, Oxford OX2 6DP

Oxford University Press is a department of the University of Oxford.
It furthers the University's objective of excellence in research, scholarship,
and education by publishing worldwide in

Oxford New York

Athens Auckland Bangkok Bogotá Buenos Aires Cape-Town
Chennai Dar-es-Salaam Delhi Florence Hong-Kong Istanbul Karachi
Kolkata Kuala-Lumpur Madrid Melbourne Mexico-City Mumbai Nairobi
Paris São-Paulo Shanghai Singapore Taipei Tokyo Toronto Warsaw

with associated companies in Berlin Ibadan

Oxford is a registered trade mark of Oxford University Press
in the UK and in certain other countries

Published in the United States
by Oxford University Press Inc., New York

© Oxford University Press, 2011

British Library Cataloguing in Publication Data

Data available

Library of Congress Cataloging in Publication Data
Data available

Typeset in Minion by Cenveo, Bangalore, India
Printed and bound by CPI Group (UK) Ltd,
Croydon, CR0 4YY

ISBN 978-0-19-959929-5

10 9 8 7 6 5 4 3 2 1

Foreword

Professor Lukas Radbruch, President of the EAPC

The European Association for Palliative Care (EAPC) has recently formulated its new mission statement: The EAPC brings together many voices to forge a vision of excellence in palliative care that meets the needs of patients and their families. It strives to develop and promote palliative care in Europe through information, education and research using multi-professional collaboration, while engaging with stakeholders at all levels.

This mission necessitates a multi-professional and interdisciplinary approach, in accordance with the holistic definition of palliative care. However, palliative care often focuses on the medical and nursing care of the individual patient. Astonishing advances have been made in pain relief and symptom management, and patients with advanced cancer are offered almost routinely counselling and support from palliative care services. From the United Kingdom, where Cicely Saunders had set down the seeds with the opening of St Christopher's Hospice in 1967, hospice and palliative care has spread to many other countries in the world. With many subsequent steps, leading up to the National End of Life strategy that again established a marker for other European countries, the United Kingdom has stayed in the lead of palliative care development in Europe. In an EAPC attempt to compare the stage of palliative care in European countries, the United Kingdom has been used as the gold standard, setting the state of palliative care there at 100 per cent.

However, although in the UK and in some other countries the development has reached an impressive stage, and the provision of palliative care has reached or is approaching proper coverage in some countries, there is still the worrying impression that some groups of patients are not in the focus of vision.

In most countries palliative care is linked closely to cancer care, and patients with other life-threatening diseases find it much harder to access palliative care. This has even raised the question, whether palliative care is for cancer patients only, and similar care for non-cancer patients would have to be named differently. Even though the EAPC strongly advocates 'palliative care' as the common term for all patients with life-threatening diseases, this discussion demonstrates that some patient groups will find it easier to access adequate palliative care.

Older people are coming only slowly within the focus of palliative care. They may suffer from cancer, but also from other diseases. Disease trajectories may be much slower in non-cancer patients, and palliative care staff may find it difficult to adjust to different needs in these patients. Similarly, dementia is recognized as a specific field for palliative care, requiring a different set of skills than for cancer patients.

Assessment and treatment have to adapt to the cognitive impairments. More important, palliative care for older people as well as for patients with dementia also presents major organizational challenges. What is the best setting to treat these patients? Specialized palliative care units may find it hard to cater for the needs of these patients. Specialized geriatric and dementia services are rare in most countries in Europe. These patients are often cared for in nursing homes, but the standard of care in nursing homes may be insufficient for them, and the economic circumstances of nursing homes often do not allow for adequate expansion of palliative care.

Social and ethnic differences also seem to play a role, even in countries with highly developed social security systems that should ensure that everybody who needs palliative care can access it. This seems to be less true not only for the aged, but also for specific groups such as travellers or homeless people. Little is known about the needs of these groups, and concepts for the provision of palliative care for them are lacking.

The book presented here closes the gap and describes not only general social issues such as poverty, ethnicity, and gender, but also provides guidance for palliative care in specific groups, going from specific needs to treatment issues to models of care for these groups. However, the strongest point of the book is not to provide a textbook approach, but rather to point at the weak spots in the fabric of palliative care. Thus it initiates and fuels the discussion on how to improve in these areas. This discussion is needed in many European countries, where palliative care has gone past the pioneer stage. Palliative care professionals, who have to take care of patients with particular needs and policy planners, who have to acknowledge these needs and have to set up services accordingly, may find this book particularly helpful for their work.

The discussion on how to improve the weak spots of palliative care contributes directly to the mission of the EAPC. Only with this discussion can we forge a vision of palliative care that meets the needs of all patients and their families. The editors have to be congratulated on the compilation of such a comprehensive review of the social differences and the influence they have on the provision of palliative care.

Contents

List of Contributors

Katherine Cox
Integrative Psychotherapist,
Twickenham, UK

Nigel G. J. Dodds
Community Nurse Manager,
St Christopher's Hospice, London, UK

Murna Downs
Head, Bradford Dementia Group,
Division of Dementia Studies,
School of Health Studies,
University of Bradford, UK

Chris Farnham
Consultant in Palliative Medicine,
Hospice of St John and St Elizabeth,
London, UK

Anthony C. Gatrell
Dean, School of Health and Medicine,
Lancaster University, UK

Anne Grinyer
Division of Health Research,
School of Health & Medicine,
Lancaster University, UK

Barbara Hanratty
Senior Lecturer in Population and
Community Health,
University of Liverpool, UK

Max Henderson
Clinical Senior Lecturer in
Epidemiological & Occupational
Psychiatry, Institute of Psychiatry,
King's College London, UK

Jo Hockley
Nurse Consultant,
St Christopher's Hospice, London, UK

Louise Holmes
Research Assistant,
University of Liverpool, UK

Glennys Howarth
Professor, Faculty of Health,
University of Plymouth, UK

Louise Jones
Head, Marie Curie Palliative Care
Research Unit, Research Department
of Mental Health Sciences,
University College London, UK

Orla Keegan
Head of Education,
Research and Bereavement Services,
Irish Hospice Foundation,
Dublin, Ireland

Jonathan Koffman
Senior Lecturer in Palliative Care,
King's College London,
Department of Palliative Care,
Policy and Rehabilitation,
Cicely Saunders Institute,
London, UK

May McCreaddie
Lecturer, School of Nursing,
Midwifery and Health,
University of Stirling, UK

Regina McQuillan
Consultant in Palliative Medicine,
St Francis Hospice,
Dublin, Ireland

Barbara Monroe
Chief Executive, St Christopher's
Hospice, London, UK

Caroline Nicholson
Post Doctoral Research Fellow,
National Nursing Research Unit,
Florence Nightingale School of
Nursing & Midwifery, King's College
London, UK

David Oliviere
Director of Education and Training,
St Christopher's Hospice, London, UK

Malcolm Payne
Adviser, Policy and Development,
St Christopher's Hospice, London, UK

Sheila Payne
Professor, School of Health and
Medicine, Lancaster University, UK

Annabel Price
Clinical Lecturer in Palliative Care
Liaison Psychiatry, Institute of
Psychiatry, King's College London, UK

Lukas Radbruch
President of the European Association
for Palliative Medicine;
Chair of Palliative Medicine,
Department of Palliative Medicine,
University Hospital Bonn, Germany

Mike Richards
National Cancer Director, National
Cancer Action Team, London, UK

Heather Richardson
Clinical Director, St Joseph's Hospice,
London, UK

Kelli I. Stajduhar
Associate Professor, School of Nursing
and Centre on Ageing,
University of Victoria, Canada

Carol Thomas
Professor of Sociology,
Division of Health Research,
Lancaster University, UK

Irene Tuffrey-Wijne
Senior Research Fellow,
St George's University of London, UK

Mary Turner
Research Fellow,
Lancaster University, UK

Part 1

Chapter 1

Introduction: Social differences— the challenge for palliative care

Barbara Monroe, David Oliviere, and Sheila Payne

Responsiveness to individual need and circumstance and attention to issues of cultural sensitivity has been at the heart of palliative care from its inception. This book has been conceived out of a conviction that everyone approaching the end of their life should have access to good support, whoever they are, wherever they live, and whatever their circumstances. Central to achieving this aim is a recognition of the importance of the social aspects of palliative care. If the demands of social justice are to be met there must be a shift in understanding that enlarges the current predominantly individually based model to include an analysis of, and action in response to, structural inequalities. These relate to legal, political, and economic considerations in different societies. History also plays a role in shaping communities and health care policies, which in turn impact on the resources and quality of services available to dying individuals and those close to them. As Dodds' chapter in this book, on refugees and asylum seekers, reminds us, many individuals and communities have experienced histories of injustice and oppression which do not disappear when terminal illness, death and bereavement become part of their lives.

Differences across societies are reflected in patterns of illness and inequalities experienced by individuals, families, and communities throughout life. They are also present in their dying. Using the UK as an example, the publication of the Marmot Review, 'Fairer Society, Healthy Lives', in 2010 drew a stark picture of health inequalities in England. It concluded that, 'people with a higher socioeconomic position in society have a greater array of life chances and more opportunities to lead a flourishing life. They also have better health' (Marmot, 2010). Crudely speaking, the wealthier you are, the healthier you are. The gap between rich and poor in the UK now means that the poor are twice as likely to die before reaching the age of 65 than the most affluent. That these inequalities exist in a society recently ranked top in the delivery of end of life care (Economist Intelligence Unit, 2010) must be a source of concern.

This book analyses the wide range of social factors and differences which can affect access to services, assessment, interventions and individual and family experience as death approaches. The first part addresses wider contextual issues; the second describes some of the groups in our societies which still lack access to good palliative care. (See Figure 1.1.)

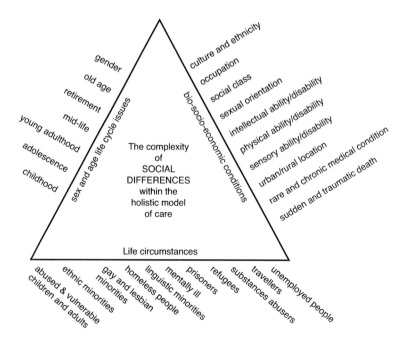

Fig. 1.1 Framework of Social Differences.

The roll call of the disadvantaged remains largely unchanged since the first edition of this book, when we commented that 'well-meaning attempts to protect children continue to leave them ignored and isolated as they face bereavement; people with learning disabilities are sometimes denied information; prisoners with advanced illnesses often end their lives in far from adequate medical conditions, minority ethnic communities still have unequal access to good care; the needs of refugees and asylum seekers with traumatic past experiences often remain invisible. Add to these examples patients with particular health conditions, such as dementia, psychiatric illness, or non-malignant illness; those who are in a variety of specific social circumstances, for example, those at risk of abuse or who abuse substances; and the different identities based on gender, sexuality, age, class, ability; and a huge multiplicity of need based on social differences is demonstrated. The challenge for palliative care providers and commissioners is not only discerning and responding to the needs and wants of these groups, but also recognizing the variation within the groups themselves.'

A thread running throughout this book, and all of our lives and deaths, is gender. As Howarth reminds us in her chapter, gender cuts across all class and ethnic divisions. Dying is a gendered experience; the vast majority of the health and social care workforce are female. The gender of individuals can determine the perception of them by others and by themselves. The way men and women experience roles, expectations, socialization, and conditioning is diverse and will affect their experiences of illness, death, and bereavement. Gender itself is mediated by culture, geography, generation, and class. Certain characteristics cluster to form multiple sources of inequity, such as for single or widowed older women living in poverty.

Some inequalities are so embedded in our systems and accepted norms that they have escaped the spotlight in discussions of disadvantage and exclusion. Recognition of ageist assumptions and the inadequate response to the needs of older people is a good example. It is only recently that the realities of the sheer scale of the increasing numbers and proportion of older people in many Western societies has led to a focus on the deficiencies in the end of life care of many of them and the education and support needs of the care home sector, which in the UK has three times as many beds as the National Health Service. Hospices should not feel sanguine about their own services; a British study on cancer inequalities indicated that the proportion of people dying with cancer at home or in a hospice decreases with age; one-third of people under 65 with cancer die in a hospice compared with 2 per cent of those over the age of 85 (National Cancer Equality Initiative, 2010). A global recession, added to ageing populations, means that every society has to make complex, rational, yet pragmatic decisions that translate the rhetoric of progress and choice and the realities of health economics into appropriate service delivery for all groups and communities of the dying. The pursuit of excellence for all may be unattainable; perhaps we should strive instead for 'good enough' services delivered with attention to dignity and respect.

This book reflects on the changing nature of information and the demands of good communication. Data are not information; they need interpretation and management and here culture is an important filter. We quote again from the introduction to the first edition about challenges that remain apposite. 'Much of the literature and basic professional assumptions of palliative care are defined by mainstream attitudes about death. Despite our avowed cultural sensitivity, a "heroic script" (Seale, 1995; Walter, 1999) defines much of what we do with an insistence on independence, autonomy, and disclosure. How do we provide appropriate care for minority ethnic and religious groups which are diverse within themselves? What training for professionals will help us to examine our own prejudices and assumptions, and to work appropriately with the conflicts that arise as we work, for example, with groups that favour patriarchal decision-making, or where informed consent for women seems a long way off? What roles should context and relativism properly play in our decision-making? How should we respond to Gunaratnam's (1997) suggestion that our vaunted cultural sensitivity should give way to a more assertive agenda of race equality?'

Richardson's and Koffman's description in this book of a project to improve the confidence of black and minority ethnic communities in utilizing and gaining a say in developing the services of a London hospice indicates the human and financial costs of effective responsiveness. As communities become increasingly diverse many minorities feel excluded from mainstream services. Listening to users' narratives can assist us to challenge our own perceptions and to recognize how the processes of engagement and interaction need to empower before effective care can be delivered.

Advances in palliative care treatments and symptom control run the risk of prompting the development of ever more standardzed models of service delivery designed to fit the needs of a norm based on our largely unchallenged assumptions. In the UK the advent of personal health care budgets and a trumpeted 'Information Revolution' (Department of Health, 2010), with its emphasis on allowing users to compare services and outcomes, may serve to improve the position of the articulate and well networked dying whilst further diminishing opportunities for the vulnerable and less articulate who often require significant, potentially costly, well-coordinated and individualized support to achieve access. In a cash strapped environment the likelihood of 'top up' payments for universal health and social care services will create further inequalities. There are challenges here for those countries with largely voluntary sector hospices and their ethos and practice. They will need to consider the changing nature of their relationship with individual patients who may wish to purchase services at a 'price' set by the organization, whilst others are unable to do so. The hospice 'movement' in the UK and elsewhere has lobbied hard for its own funding, perhaps less so on issues of social justice. One of the challenges raised by this book is for practitioners to think more widely and more sensitively about the very different settings in which end of life care is, should, or will be delivered. The established practices associated with hospice led palliative care are not appropriate everywhere and for all populations, as Nicholson and Hockley remind us in their chapter on frail, older people. Keegan's chapter on bereavement also reminds us that established assumptions about grief and bereavement care have served to disenfranchize many and that the focus on individual therapy has neglected the value of community development approaches. Research agendas need to focus on the development of a setting appropriate evidence base.

This book makes it clear that a focus on individual welfare alone cannot meet global aspirations for good end of life care. Field, writing in 2000, emphasized that for dying individuals 'the meaning, experience, and expression of their terminal illness is shaped and influenced by the communities within which they live. The social fabric of their lives is central to how they make sense of their illness experiences, the meanings they draw upon to understand these, and the range of resources they can call upon to help them manage them'. Money alone cannot ensure coverage. The largely volunteer-based palliative care service in Kerala is an inspiring example of how good care can reach all, even on a tiny budget, when communities and professionals mobilize together (Kumar, 2007). The editors believe that an international perspective is vital if we are to meet the challenges facing the provision of end of life care, and share mutual learning.

In a recent study of depression in the palliative care population, which had the largest sample size yet achieved in the UK, low social support emerged as the most significant risk factor for non-remission of depression (Goodwin et al., 2011). This emphasizes the importance of fostering social relationships, particularly at the end of life when patients and their families may find themselves severed from work and friendship links. Support to re-establish lost relationships may be vital as the chapter on homeless individuals suggests. Payne (Malcolm) describes 'social capital' as the 'power that we gain by having wide and supportive networks of relationships'. We all need to give as well as to receive and this is nowhere more important than at the end of life. Payne also reminds us that even government-backed approaches to respond to 'social exclusion' can in themselves become discriminatory. Palliative care services need to be aware of their responsibility to promote social cohesion through education and positive action. Growing need and dwindling resources, both financial and professional, make a health promotion approach all the more important so that communities themselves can respond sensitively and appropriately to the diverse needs of dying and bereaved individuals. New forms of volunteer development and engagement will be needed to meet the demands of an ageing population living with multiple chronic conditions, alongside significant changes in a wide variety of family structures.

Professionals are not immune to the stereotypes of the population. Some patients' inability to give expected forms of positive feedback (for example asylum seekers, those with dementia, intellectual disabilities, or significant mental health problems) may make them appear 'unrewarding' as potential recipients of mainstream palliative care services. As we asked in the previous volume, 'are we offering people equal access to "our" services, or to the ones *they* want and need?' This book aims to provide some practical suggestions for service improvement but asks more questions than it offers solutions. This seems an appropriate stance for a mature sector facing ever growing challenges. More must be achieved with less and there are important conversations ahead about how professionals can achieve collaborative partnerships with communities, patients and those close to them so that death can be restored to its proper place as a natural part of life. It would be a tragedy if the last century's important focus on, and achievements in pursuit of cure, left us haunted by the spectre of endlessly added years of poor quality existence.

References

Department of Health (2010). *Liberating the NHS: An information revolution.* London: Department of Health Publications.

Economist Intelligence Unit (2010). *The Quality of Death: Ranking end of life care across the world.* London: EIU.

Field, D. (2000). *What do we mean by 'psychosocial'?* Briefing No. 4, March. London: National Council for Hospice and Specialist Palliative Care Services.

Goodwin, L., Lee, W., Price, A., Rayner, L., Monroe, B., Sykes, N., et al. (2011). Predictors of non-remission of depression in a palliative care population. Accepted for publication by *Palliative Medicine.*

Gunaratnam, Y. (1997). Culture is not enough: A critique of multi-culturalism in palliative care. In: Field, D., Hockey, J., and Small, N. (eds), *Death, Gender and Ethnicity.* London: Routledge.

Kumar, S. (2007). Kerala, India: A regional community based palliative care model. *Journal of Pain and Symptom Management,* **33**(5): 623–7.

Marmot, M. (2010). The Marmot Review. *Fair Society, Healthy Lives. Strategic Review of Health Inequalities in England post-2010.* London: The Marmot Review. www.ucl.ac.nh/marmotreview. Accessed 6/1/11.

National Cancer Equality Initiative. (2010). *Reducing Cancer Inequality: Evidence, progress and making it happen.* London: National Cancer Action Team, Department of Health.

Seale, C. (1995). Heroic death. *Sociology,* **29**(4): 597–613.

Walter, T. (1999). *On Bereavement: The culture of grief.* Buckingham, UK: Open University Press.

Chapter 2

The emergence of new forms of dying in contemporary societies

Glennys Howarth

Introduction

It is often suggested that people are dying from the moment they are born. Dying, however, is more commonly discussed in the context of disease or illness, whether the onset is sudden and acute with a rapid trajectory or the slow and frequently debilitating decline of old age. There are essentially two elements to dying: the biological and the social. Biologically speaking, dying takes places as the tissues and organs cease to function and death can occur within minutes of the beginning of the process. In social terms, dying usually takes considerably longer and, as Kellehear (2007: 2) argues, this is the conscious dying that we observe when, 'we live in that urgent space created by the *awareness*, that death is soon to engulf us', or those we love and care for.

The way in which dying is experienced is impacted by social structural factors such as socio-economic status, ethnicity, and gender. It is important in identifying these factors to note that these are not mutually exclusive categories and it is difficult to distinguish the effect of social class from that of ethnicity, and to recognize that gender cuts across all class and ethnic divisions. That said, socio-economic status influences life experiences, such as housing, education, occupation, peer group, geographical location, and access to public and private resources, all of which have a bearing on the way in which health and illness, and consequently dying, are experienced. For example, a lower life expectancy is associated with people in the lowest socio-economic group; in the UK in the years 1992–6 men in Social Class I could expect to live, on average, nine and a half years longer than those in Social Class V (Hattersley, 1999). This reduced life expectancy is linked to poor living conditions, environmental hazards, and the risk of dying in sudden or violent circumstance, for example, in workplace accidents and from related diseases such as asbestosis. These conditions also negatively impact on minority ethnic groups, particularly those living in poor inner city areas where levels of health and life expectancy rates may be more characteristic of those found in a poor developing nation (Murray, 2000).

This chapter focuses on the social aspects of dying and the way in which these have changed across historical periods in Western societies. It begins with an examination of dying as a social relationship and explores how the experience or understanding of dying has changed across time and within different communities. The turn from religious to medical authority is considered within a discussion of changing mores, *ars moriendi*, and expectations about the nature and timing of the 'good death'. There will be a discussion of physical illnesses and diseases that led to death in previous periods followed by an examination of more contemporary forms of dying. Here, following the progress of public health reforms and medical technology, the significance of the change from acute infectious diseases to more chronic disabling illnesses will be highlighted, together with the impact this has on dying in modern societies.

In the context of care of the dying, this role has historically been perceived as a family or community responsibility but is now predominantly seen in terms of service provision with some people more privileged than others in their ability to access care. This section of the chapter will engage with issues of inequality and discrimination, powerlessness, vulnerability and stigma.

The final section of the chapter will set the discussion in the context of Kellehear's (2007) theory of the social ages of dying and will consider dying in contemporary societies, highlighting popular expectations and choices—a major distinction between dying in previous era and dying today. Dying has now been tempered by pain-relieving drugs, therapies and technologies that, to some extent and in some cases, can provide a measure of control over the timing of death. Moreover, where once dying was seen as inevitable and determined by God or fate, today people are frequently not only able to defer dying due to advances in medical technology such as organ transplantation, but are also, in some situations and countries, able to choose when to die, for example, in the case of euthanasia. The chapter concludes with some remarks about the implications of these new conditions of dying in terms of resources and service provision.

Dying as a social relationship

It is worth noting here that in focusing on the social characteristics of dying, the emphasis is on dying as a social relationship. Dying involves awareness, either on the part of the individual themselves or the awareness of observers. The extent to which the dying person participates in the process depends on the degree of their awareness and their dying trajectory—a long, drawn out terminal illness as distinct from the dying that takes places in the minutes or moments following a sudden, traumatic event such as a fatal car crash. Yet, even when the dying person is unaware of their terminal state, others around them may know that death is close and be able to engage with the dying process. Thus, the majority of forms of dying involve the participation of others and engage in social relationships with survivors or professionals.

In the context of what Kellehear (2007) refers to as 'managed dying' (which will be discussed later in the chapter), Glaser and Strauss (1965) argue that this is a social relationship that involves a series of status passages wherein the dying person transits through a number of different periods or events which provide cues to observers as to where they are located along the journey. In an institutional setting, observers include family, medical personnel, health professionals, and care staff, who all 'engage in trying to ascertain where he [*sic*] is, in order to guide their own behaviour' (Glaser and Strauss, 1965: 50). Although Glaser and Strauss were specifically referring to dying in the twentieth century, this search for signs of where the dying person is located in the process is common across time and cultures. To illustrate this we will consider dying through history in Western societies. This will be discussed in the context of Omran's (1971) theory of 'epidemiological transitions'.

Historical depictions of dying in Western societies

The theory of epidemiological transitions

Omran's (1971) theory of epidemiological transitions provides a framework for an initial understanding of changes to the nature of dying within Western societies. Accordingly, there are three stages of transition that describe the nature of illness, dying and death and through which, he argued, all societies must pass. The stages are self-explanatory, the first being the age of pestilence and famine, the second an age of receding pandemics when societies are more able to combat infectious diseases, and the third is the age of degenerative diseases within which people live extended lives but accompanied by longer periods of chronic illness and disability at the end of life. Although Omran's theory has been criticized for assuming a progression from one stage to another (Howarth, 2009) it does provide a framework for an account of the epidemiological conditions prevalent at different historical periods and which have affected the way in which dying is experienced.

The age of pestilence and famine: Europe in the Middle Ages

Europe, during the Middle Ages, was primarily comprised of agricultural or rural societies with a number of urban centres. These were societies at the mercy of pandemics, natural disasters, famine and violent death. In an age where there was little understanding of the nature of disease and infection, diseases such as smallpox, cholera, and plague ran rife and decimated populations throughout Europe. For example, the Black Death of the 1340s is estimated to have killed somewhere between 25 and 50 million people—death usually occurring within a few days of the first appearance of symptoms. In these pre-industrial societies famine was also prevalent and in agrarian communities that relied for survival on successful harvests, starvation was a constant threat. Dying from malnutrition is a relatively slow process that takes place across weeks or months with the individual becoming weaker and critically ill as death approaches. Thus, whilst many of the causes of death resulted in a truncated period between the onset of illness and final demise, others, such as smallpox and starvation had a longer gestation and the person, aware that death was approaching, would have had time to reflect on life and make preparations for death.

Ariès (1981), whose classic study of dying has for decades structured our understanding of death across historical periods in Western societies, depicts dying in this period as an aware dying that was considered to be inevitable, determined by God, and which involved the dying person attempting to experience a good death by making both this world and otherworld preparations. Knowing that death is near allows for the opportunity to make decisions about how to dispose of personal effects and on whom to bestow any remaining wealth. It also prompts consideration of dealing with any unfinished business, such as healing any family rifts or making amends for acts or behaviour regretted during life. This concern to deal with earthly matters was complimented by a pressing need to ensure that the soul was fully prepared for the next life. The *ars moriendi* were popular during this time and were Christian texts that, used together with the services of a priest, provided information on the appropriate religious rituals designed to successfully guide the dying person into the afterlife.

It is probably safe to say, though, that these sorts of preparations would have been largely available only to the elite classes who had possessions to pass on to others, time to reflect on their deathbeds, and priests available to assist with religious rituals. The majority of poor peasant or urban dwellers would not have had such luxuries and their care and ritual preparation would most likely have involved family, friends, and neighbours in the community. This is not to suggest a necessarily poorer quality of dying, simply that their dying experiences and their social relationships at that time would probably have been less managed, with little professional assistance and guidance. Although a priest would have been sought near the very end of life, the experience would probably have been more participatory, being involved in everyday routines and cared for according to age-old traditions and rituals.

The age of receding pandemics

As European societies became more industrialized in the eighteenth and nineteenth centuries, and urban centres grew both in size and significance, rural communities contracted and with that the familiar knowledge of signs, awareness and rituals around dying were lost or transformed. As Kellehear suggests, the peasant understanding of the cyclical harmony and balance in nature, the 'round of time' (2007: 87) that is so much a feature of the work of contemporary novelists such as Thomas Hardy, nostalgically regretting the passing of rural traditions and proximity to nature, was, to a large extent, lost in the move to the towns and cities with the emphasis on industry and business and, for the poorer classes, the poverty and squalor of crowded urban slum dwelling. Although understanding of the causes and successful treatment of infection continued to evade the blossoming medical profession, it was during this period that public health strategies slowly began to impact on the health of nations. By the end of the nineteenth century there was a greater understanding of nutrition, public health, and sanitation, and this combination resulted in a significant decline in infant mortality rates and longevity more generally. This change to life expectancy, however, impacted differentially according to social class, for example, life expectancy for working-class people did not begin to increase for at least 30 years after that for higher social strata (Mitchison, 1977).

Nevertheless, infectious diseases continued to plague the populations of Europe and North American and one of the biggest killers of the late eighteenth and nineteenth centuries in both rural and urban communities was tuberculosis (TB), or consumption as it was frequently referred to. Although TB has been around for centuries, during the seventeenth and eighteenth centuries it is thought to have been responsible for 25 per cent of all the deaths in Europe. One primary reason for this high mortality rate was the fact that it was not until 1882 that Robert Koch identified it as an infectious disease, and 1946 when the first antibiotic was introduced to combat the illness. During the nineteenth century consumption, which was usually fatal, was commonly viewed among the middle-class intellectual and artistic community through the lens of the Romantic sensibilities of the day with the disease thought to bestow upon sufferers a heightened sensitivity to art and literature. Although the disease was feared, those dying of consumption were depicted as doing so gracefully, slowly 'fading away, transcending their corporeal body, their immortal soul shining through' (Manoli-Skocay, 2003: 1). By the end of the nineteenth century and into the early twentieth century, however (possibly as a consequence of heightened popular expectations of cure and extended life expectancy), tuberculosis had lost its romantic connotations and came to be seen as an infectious disease of the poorer classes, linked to urban poverty and poor housing and striking them down in greater numbers than their wealthier counterparts. Once the disease was demystified medically, it became stigmatized and feared. It threatened social order in that it negatively reflected both the prospect of an unpleasant dying and premature death, and also, due to the negative social conditions that gave rise to and propagated the disease, it frequently wiped out whole families who were either ignorant of its contagious nature or unable to secure the resources to isolate and care for the infected person.

In the context of Omran's theory of epidemiological transitions, the first half of the twentieth century in Western societies could more appropriately be described as an age of receding pandemics. Greater understanding of the aetiology of disease, public health reforms, and the discovery and development of antibiotics to combat infection, all combined to reduce the devastating effect of contagious diseases. From the mid-twentieth century further headway was made in the development of medical interventions and technologies that provided new hope for cures for previously fatal diseases and promised greater life expectancy. The high infant mortality rate of previous centuries was significantly reduced and by the 1930s parents in all social classes could anticipate that their children would outlive them (Mitchison, 1977).

The age of degenerative disease: contemporary society

The later decades of the century and into the twenty-first century conform to Omran's third stage of epidemiological transition, that of degenerative diseases. The five biggest killers in Western societies are now heart disease, cancer, cerebro-vascular disease (stroke), diseases of the lung, and accidents. Due to advances in medicine, medical technology and public health strategies, dying commonly occurs at an older age but the body becomes the site of disease and fragility as organs begin to wear out and thus dying is frequently a slow, degenerative process. As people live longer the incidence of degenerative diseases has amplified and acute illness and relatively brief dying trajectories have been replaced by extended periods of chronic illness and disability (Ashby, 2009). Thus longevity has been achieved at a cost as the number of years of poor health at the end of life has increased and this has led to the question of the appropriate balance between quantity and quality of life.

In Western societies that prize autonomy and independence, an increasing health risk is that of dementia; a disease that gradually leads to the loss of self, beginning with impairment of rational thought and reasoning power and eventually loss of instinctive and voluntary responses. It is estimated that the disease currently affects 35 per cent of people over the age of 90 (Brown and Hillam, 2004), and it is predicted that by 2020, 29 million people world-wide will be living with dementia.

Although a global disease, HIV/AIDS is a modern pandemic that currently affects around 40 million people world-wide and has resulted in over 25 million deaths. The burden of disease is greatest in Africa and south-east Asia, where poverty and social stigma compound the physical indignities of the illness. In Western societies AIDS has been largely associated with homosexual sexual activity and drug use and this has resulted in considerable social stigma for those who have contracted it. AIDS thus came to be viewed as a moral issue; the dying experience influenced by the cultural context in which moral judgements are made about the terminally ill person. People with HIV and a weakened immune system are more susceptible to other infectious disease and the illness has given rise to a resurgence of TB. Whilst the majority of cases of this secondary infection are found in the developing world, TB has once again become a concern for industrial societies thus undermining Omran's theory of progression through his stages of epidemiological transition.

The good death and care of the dying

No description of forms of dying in Europe would be complete without a discussion of the 'good death'. The good death is one that is managed according to socially pre-scribed processes. It is constructed through a process of cultural negotiation and according to contemporary mores and values. As Sontag (1978) observes, metaphors of illness and disease reflect moral judgements associated with particular causes of dying and this analysis can be extended to include judgements surrounding the manner in which people die. Sudden, violent death, for example, is more likely to be experienced by those marginal to mainstream society—the very poor and ethnic and religious minorities. These are people with less power and fewer resources available to them and, in many cases, with a cultural history of deference to authority that brings with it a reli-ance on, and trust in those deemed to have greater knowledge. Their inability to effect control and to be involved in end of life decision-making is compounded by their lack of access to information and their social exclusion (Strange, 2009).

Historically, the good death has been associated with religious preparations for the next life. It is usually depicted as a process in which the person, aware that they are dying, is able to finalize their business in this world and to complete spiritual tasks that will provide them safe passage into the next. It is stereotypically described, following the work of Ariès (1981), as a 'tame death' wherein the individual dies at home on their deathbed, is resigned to dying, and has family members and professionals (particularly priests) to assist them on their dying journey.

In the Middle Ages the good death was highly structured and depended primarily on religious preparation for the afterlife, framed, as it was, by Christian rituals that were performed to demonstrate that the dying person had either led a good life or was truly remorseful for their sins and ready to accept divine judgement. These rituals were undertaken at the deathbed and would continue once life had expired as family, friends and priests continued to prayer for the salvation of the soul. In Protestant post-Reformation societies, once purgatory had been outlawed, care of the dying person's soul could not continue after death, so dying became more immediately linked with biological expiration and this paved the way for the doctor, rather than the priest, to become the authority over dying.

For most of history, dying people have been cared for within the family and community. Indeed, the good death described above would have entailed a process that took place in the intimacy and domesticity of the home. In wealthier homes the deathbed is likely to have been located in a room separate from the rest of the household. As such, dying was invested 'with a definite identity and apparently locating the dying process as something removed from everyday life' (Strange, 2009: 136). In poorer households there would not have been the resources to separate the dying person and so they would have remained among the living, subject to the comings and goings of everyday life and their care undertaken without too much disruption to the household. Indeed, Strange (2005) points out that from the nineteenth century, when there was the opportunity to have the dying person relocated to a hospital, families usually preferred to keep them at home, despite the moral reprobation this caused among the middle class who commented negatively on the fact that the poor kept the dying, and the dead, within the close confines of the home (Strange, 2005; Howarth, 2007). This behaviour is hardly surprising, however, given that until the twentieth century hospitals had a reputation as, 'filthy, germ-riddled institutions where people frequently died of infections' (Schachter, 2001).

The emphasis on the good Christian death began to decline during the Victorian period, such that by the 1880s there was less concern with religious piety and more 'anxiety about the physical suffering of dying. For early and mid-Victorian Christians there must often have been some conflict between the desire to display courage in the face of suffering and the human wish to die with as little pain as possible' (Jalland, 1996: 52). The concept of the good death was also seriously compromised as a consequence of the First World War when vast numbers of men died in such a brutal fashion. The hitherto popular notion of the heroic death in war also lost its gloss and romantic appeal as recruits and civilians became aware of the real horrors of this first technological war and the manner in which soldiers died far from home in the squalor and anonymity of the front line—a far cry from the, perhaps romanticized, intimacy and domesticity of previous ideals of the good death.

From around the middle of the twentieth century institutions such as the hospital, nursing home, and residential home became locations for dying in Western societies where it was estimated that by the end of the century around 80 per cent of people died in some form of institution (Field and James, 1993). During the 1950s and 1960s, the care of dying people had become medicalized (Zola, 1972) with the struggle against death taking precedence over the notion of dying well. Hospitals, with their potential life saving technology and professional expertise became the institutions where many people died. Ironically, because death was perceived as a failure of medicine, dying people were often not only unaware that they were at the end of life but were also subjected to a range of indignities designed to extend their life. For many commentators of the period this resulted in the loss of a natural death and the experience of dying was distressing, lacking in dignity, lonely, and isolating (Illich, 1976; Kübler-Ross, 1970).

The modern hospice and palliative care movement which developed as a reaction against the poor quality of care for dying people, was dedicated to facilitating a good death, defined as one in which the person is provided with symptom management and pain control and is focused around the notion of awareness and dignity. The emphasis on holistic care of the dying person aims to control 'total pain', which incorporates physical, social, emotional and spiritual pain. In so doing, there is an assumption that physical pain may mask other forms of pain and vice versa, and so the model of care aims to alleviate distress by controlling physical pain and with it, reducing emotional and spiritual suffering. Whilst this is an admirable intention, it has been suggested that placing all forms of suffering within the remit of medicine (physical pain) effectively acts as a mechanism for extending medical control over dying and Clark (1999) has argued that the concept of 'total care' may effectively mask 'total control'.

Whatever the realities of hospice care it should be acknowledged that this form of dying is only available to a minority, around 6 per cent of dying people—usually those dying of cancer and, given the Christian ethos of a majority of hospices in Western societies, those who identify with the dominant ethnic group. Extended life expectancy leads to a substantial proportion of people now dying in long-term care facilities such as residential or nursing homes. Due to differences in mortality rates, with women living longer than men, dying in residential care for the elderly is a gendered experience. Unlike hospitals where there is the problem of medicalization, or hospices where dying people expect to receive treatment for 'total pain', the majority of residential homes for elderly people have limited medical support and the care regime tends to be focused on improving quality of life with little acknowledgement from staff that the residents are in the terminal phase of their lives. This is the form of dying that Kellehear (2007) refers to as the 'shameful death' in that it is a stigmatized dying that refuses an awareness of death and as such denies the opportunity for elderly people in residential care to participate in their dying. Furthermore, it is a dying experience that may eventually become the norm as life expectancy in Western societies continues to be extended.

Contemporary Western societies: a new form of dying?

So, what, if anything, is distinct about the nature of dying in contemporary Western societies and is there a new social form emerging? Prior to examining this question in depth let us first consider Kellehear's (2007) theoretical framework for understanding social forms of dying. Rather than linking types of dying to historical periods, in his carefully researched *Social History of Dying*, Kellehear (2007: 210) claims four 'major forms of dying [that] may be found in all times and places'. These are based on the nature of society and the epidemiological conditions therein, and result in one form of dying taking precedence over others in a particular society.

Kellehear begins his typology with Stone Age societies where death is sudden and occurs as a consequence of trauma such as accidents or animal attacks, leaving little or no opportunity for preparation or awareness. Here, he suggests, dying takes places *after*, not prior to death, and comprises a series of rituals or processes performed by survivors, most likely to prepare the dead for the journey and entry into the next life. There is no self-awareness on the part of the dying person, except in the identity constructed by the surviving group who 'give' him or her a 'dying' (2007: 25).

In the second age, the Pastoral Age of settled societies, where life becomes more stable and less mobile, people live longer than in Stone Age societies and although still frequently sudden (for example, in war or other disputes), death becomes more predictable, caused by infectious diseases and, not unusually, famine. The dying person is, therefore, more likely to be aware of his/her demise and more able to participate in preparations for death.

The third form of dying that Kellehear considers is that which is dominant in the Urban Age in which the 'managed death' comes to the fore: a death that is good by virtue of having professional services and guidance. The dying person's role as participant becomes weakened as they become a, 'site for services . . . it would be the professional 'others' who would manage our dying through 'medical investigations', 'estate management and will-making', 'psychological or spiritual interventions', or 'supportive' cancer or aged care services (2007: 145).

The final form of dying that Kellehear deals with is that of the Cosmopolitan Age. In the Cosmopolitan Age, dying is characterized by shame, the shame of stigmatized dying that occurs when life has been lived for too long—in 'overripe' old age—or when it is a result of behaviour that society finds inappropriate or immoral—for example, dying of AIDS. The features of this form of dying entail a focus on chronic illness and disability with little or no awareness or acknowledgement that dying is taking place at all, and hence, with no recognition of, or respect for the need to make preparations.

There is clear evidence of Kellehear's social ages of dying throughout this chapter where elements of the Pastoral, Urban and Cosmopolitan ages can be distinguished: the increasingly predictable dying in the rural societies of the Middle Ages, the managed dying of modernity, and the shameful dying experienced by elderly people and those dying from stigmatized diseases in contemporary societies.

What is particularly distinctive about dying in contemporary Western societies is the expectation of longevity and the heightened perception of there being choices at the end of life, the extent and range of which might be seen as reflecting the nature of dying in each of Kellehear's post-Stone-Age forms: pastoral, urban, and cosmopolitan.

There is an anticipation that everyone is entitled to live to 'a ripe old age', again in the context of the UK, for women around 83 years old and for men 80 (OECD, 2001). Death in youth or middle age is deemed to be premature with years of potential life lost, counted down from the age at which they should more reasonably have died. As Ashby remarks, 'The stunning achievements of medical science in an age of scientific optimism have led to a level of expectation in the community, which often significantly exceeds reality' (2009: 83). Health promotion strategies have also played an important role in this respect and have proved highly influential by presenting populations with a narrative of health that relies on people taking responsibility for their own health by eating a balanced diet, taking sufficient exercise, limiting alcohol intake, quitting smoking, and so on. The health promotion literature can reasonably lead people to believe that making the correct health choices will result in a long and healthy life.

In societies where medical advances have won a victory over most infectious diseases, ill health is to a large extent perceived as avoidable. So, for example, if an organ fails as a consequence of deficiency or because unhealthy life choices have been made in the past, there may be an expectation that a transplant is a life-saving possibility—despite the scarcity of organs and the strict criteria used to determine eligibility and priority status.

A further potential choice for some people is the possibility of euthanasia or physician assisted suicide if a dying person is unable or unwilling to live with a terminal illness. There is much debate about the pros and cons of euthanasia and whilst many people and interest groups are opposed to the practice on ethical, religious, or political grounds, for others, euthanasia is a form of 'good death' in that it is a method of attaining a dignified dying that ends pain and suffering whilst remaining in control of the nature and timing of death. Those against euthanasia frequently cite the need to preserve life and care for the dying and argue that the practice may become a 'slippery slope' whereby elderly, disabled, and chronically ill people will, at some point in the future, have no choice but to accept the premature termination of their lives—involuntary euthanasia. Those in favour usually emphasize the rights of the individual to take control over their dying and to enable them to die with dignity (Kuhse and Singer, 1997). The pro-euthanasia lobby is also concerned about the quality of life experienced by people, who as a consequence of medical advances may now live into late old age with incapacitating chronic illness.

Kellehear (2007) makes it clear that the forms or ages of social dying on which his theory is based are not mutually exclusive but can occur at any time and in any place according to the nature and epidemiology of society. The fragmented nature of contemporary societies lends itself to a mix of different forms of dying. For those who are able to avail themselves of palliative care, the managed death of the urban age where there is such a reliance on professionals to guide and support people through dying, is the one most likely to be experienced. There is also a popular perception in contemporary Western societies, particularly in countries such as the UK with its welfare state, that a managed dying with access to end of life services is a right rather than a privilege. For those who have lived a long life and find themselves living in a nursing or residential home, chronically disabled or demented in their dying years, the shameful death of the cosmopolitan age is the one most likely to be experienced. Yet, there are communities who continue to provide care and support to their dying members in a manner that is more akin with the pastoral age in which dying people are helped through the experience without the overriding control of medical experts. That is not to romanticize the pastoral age, particularly when it is the case that for people who are unable to access adequate or consistent services, dying may be a painful, unpleasant, and deeply traumatic experience.

In contemporary Western societies that are currently experiencing the financial impact of a global recession, and in a context in which end of life services are stretched and under increasing pressure, there is a need to acknowledge and attempt to revive, and to further stimulate, forms of dying and care that draw from a range of models. Wherever possible these should ensure high quality care but with less reliance on professional services and more recognition of the significant role that communities might play in taking greater responsibility for the care of their dying members.

References

Ariès, P. (1981). *The Hour of Our Death*. London: Allen Lane.

Ashby, M. (2009). The dying human: a perspective from palliative medicine. In A. Kellehear (ed.), *The Study of Dying: From Autonomy to Transformation*. Cambridge: Cambridge University Press.

Brown, J. and Hillam, J. (2004). *Dementia: Your Questions Answered*. London: Churchill Livingstone.

Clark, D. (1999). 'Total Pain': Disciplinary power and the body in the work of Cicely Saunders, 1958–1967. *Social Science and Medicine*, **49**: 727–36.

Field, D. and James, N. (1993). Where and how people die. In D. Clark (ed.), *The Future for Palliative Care: Issues in Policy and Practice*. Buckingham, UK: Open University Press.

Glaser, B. G. and Strauss, A. L. (1965). Temporal aspects of dying as a non-scheduled status passage. *The American Journal of Sociology*, **17**(1): 48–59.

Hattersley, L. (1999). Trends in life expectancy by social class. *Health Statistics Quarterly*, **2**: 16–24.

Howarth, G. (2007). *Death and Dying: A Sociological Introduction*. Cambridge: Polity Press.

Howarth, G. (2009). The demography of dying. In A. Kellehear (ed.), *The Study of Dying: From Autonomy to Transformation*. Cambridge: Cambridge University Press.

Illich, I. (1976). *Limits to Medicine*. London: Marion Boyars.

Jalland, P. (1996). *Death in the Victorian Family*. Oxford: Oxford University Press.

Kellehear, A. (2007). *A Social History of Dying*. Cambridge: Cambridge University Press.

Kübler-Ross, E. (1970). *On Death and Dying*. New York: Macmillan.

Kuhse, H. and Singer, P. (1997). From the Editors: Bob Dent's decision. *Bioethics*, **11**(1): 3–5.

Manoli-Skocay, C. (2003). A gentle death: Tuberculosis in 19th century Concord. *The Concord Magazine*, Winter: 1–5.

Mitichison, R. (1977). *British Population Change Since 1860*. London: Macmillan.

Murray, C. (2000). WHO issues new health life expectancy rankings: Japan number one in new 'healthy life' system. World Health Organization press release, Washington DC and Geneva, 4 June.

OECD. (2001). *Society at a Glance: OECD Social Indicators*. Paris: CI.

Omran, A. R. (1971). The epidemiological transition: A theory of the epidemiology of population change. *Millbank Memorial Fund Quarterley*, **49**(4): 509–38.

Schachter, S. R. (2001). Hospitals. In G. Howarth and O. Leaman (eds), *Encyclopedia of Death and Dying*. London: Routledge.

Sontag, S. (1978). *Illness as Metaphor*. New York: Farrar, Straus & Giroux.

Strange, J.-M. (2005). *Death, Grief and Poverty in Britain, 1870–1914*. Cambridge: Cambridge University Press.

Strange, J.-M. (2009). Historical approaches to dying. In A. Kellehear (ed.), *The Study of Dying: From Autonomy to Transformation*. Cambridge: Cambridge University Press.

Zola, I. K. (1972). Medicine as an institution of social control. *Sociological Review*, **20**: 487–504.

Chapter 3

Social inequality in dying

Barbara Hanratty and Louise Holmes

Introduction

Watching a peaceful death of a human being reminds us of a falling star; one of a million lights in a vast sky that flares up for a brief moment only to disappear into the endless night forever. Kubler-Ross

Socio-economic inequalities in health are an unacceptable yet enduring aspect of twenty-first-century life. Death may be no respecter of wealth, but across the life course, disadvantage in material circumstances goes hand in hand with poor health status and access to health services. In recent years, health and longevity have improved overall. Global average life expectancy has risen from around 30 years in 1800, to 67 years today (Riley, 2001). With approximately 134 million births and 57 million deaths each year, the world population is expected to reach 9 billion by 2050. Much of this increase will take place in low-income countries, where the number of people aged over 60 years is forecast to rise from 473 million in 2009 to 1.6 billion in 2050 (United Nations, 2010). This picture of global ageing conceals stark contrasts in life chances, both between and within countries. A citizen of the USA lives, on average, for 78 years, 40 years longer than a typical Zambian. But a homeless man in a North American city can expect to live for between 34 and 47 years, similar to the lifespan of a man in the Cameroon. Such inequalities in life expectancy and health, by social position, geographical location, ethnicity, or gender represent one of the most important public health challenges.

Tackling the social causes of poor health and avoidable health inequalities is an urgent priority, but equally important, in the drive to produce equitable health experiences and outcomes, is to consider how the consequences of poor health vary with social position. There are many reasons why the distribution of health care needs at the end of life might vary with socio-economic status. The uneven distribution of illness is well documented. Whether individual measures of socio-economic status such as occupation or income are used, or area based indices derived from census data, the less well-off in societies are consistently shown to experience more chronic illness and die at a younger age. As well as experiencing more disease, poorer people also have greater severity of illness. Deprivation will exert a direct effect, but access to health services is also thought to be a factor. Some sections of the population: minority ethnic groups, older adults as well as lower socio-economic groups, may all experience problems in obtaining access to health care. An equitable welfare system would provide services according to care needs, and that may mean that people living in disadvantaged circumstances should have greater share of resources. But is this ever the case? This chapter presents an overview of what we currently know about social inequalities in the experience of dying. A review of existing evidence for social variation in premature mortality, cause and place of death, is followed by consideration of how access to end of life care services may differ with social position. It concludes with a discussion of how policies and funding can and should influence inequalities in end of life experiences, highlighting areas for future research and advocacy.

Premature mortality

Relative disadvantage plays an important part in determining life expectancy. A poor person in a rich country cannot expect to live as long as countrymen who are better off, whilst people in poor countries will, on average, have shorter lives than those in higher income countries. Children under 15 years account for almost half (46%) of deaths in Africa, one-quarter (24%) in South-east Asia, but only 1% in high-income countries. In low-income countries fewer than one-quarter of the population reach the age of 70 whereas more than three-quarters of people in high-income countries live beyond this age. Eighty-four per cent of deaths in high-income countries are amongst people aged more than 60 years; the comparable figure for Africa is 20%. Being a poor resident of a high-income country is also associated with shorter lifespan. In England and Wales, for example, men in unskilled occupations are almost three times more likely to die before the age of 65 years, compared to men in managerial jobs (Office for National Statistics, 2010). There is a similar socio-economic gradient in premature female mortality, with a 2.6-fold difference between the lowest and highest socio-economic categories (ONS, 2010).

Non-communicable diseases, such as cancer and cardiovascular disorders are responsible for 60% of deaths worldwide. Communicable, maternal, perinatal, and nutritional conditions together account for 30% of deaths, whilst 10% are secondary to injuries. Beneath this overarching picture, there are striking differences in causes of death between rich and poor countries. Infectious diseases are responsible for half of all deaths in childhood, most of which occur in low-income countries. There, 1 in 4 of all deaths are attributed to infectious diseases, whereas the figure for higher income countries is only 3.8%. HIV/AIDS is the leading cause of adult mortality (15–59 years old) in Africa, whereas cardiovascular diseases and injuries are the most common cause of death amongst European men in this age group (2.5 per 1,000 adults). Injuries kill more adult men in Latin America and the Caribbean (1.6 per 1,000 men) than any other causes, and road traffic accidents occur six times more often in low and middle income countries compared to high-income countries.

In England and Wales, almost two-thirds of premature mortality in males is attributed to cancers and circulatory diseases, with the steepest socio-economic gradient seen with circulatory diseases (ONS, 2010). Cardiovascular disease causes 1 in 3 deaths worldwide each year. Initially a disease of affluent countries, it is now a growing problem in developing economies, and socio-economic gradients in the incidence and mortality from cardiovascular disease are consistent across different populations and countries.

The picture is less clear-cut for cancer deaths. Total cancer mortality rates are lower amongst men with higher educational qualifications, but that is not true for all cancer sites. Men with lung cancer from the lowest socio-economic category are nearly four times more likely to die prematurely than men in the highest group. For women, the social gradient in cancer mortality is less steep, and absent in certain areas, such as Slovenia and parts of Spain (Faggiano et al., 1997; Strand et al., 2007). Such a lack of consistency in the social gradient of cancer deaths is perhaps not surprising, as cancer is not a single condition and cancers at different sites have different risk factors, illness courses and responses to treatment.

Future trends in global mortality

In the coming decades, increases in the size and age of populations are likely to have a significant influence on patterns of mortality. At present, around 2 in 3 deaths in England and Wales are amongst people aged over 75 years. By 2030, 4 in 10 decedents will be aged at least 85 years. This picture can be seen across Europe, North America and other high-income countries. As people live longer and fertility declines, the proportion of older adults in the population will go on rising. By 2030, 1 in 5 citizens of more than 55 countries will be over 65 years. World-wide, the proportion of deaths attributed to non-communicable diseases is expected to rise. Cancer deaths are predicted to increase from 7.4 million in 2004 to 11.8 million in 2030. A similar rise in cardiovascular deaths is expected, from 17.1 million in 2004 to 23.4 million in 2030. Increasing car ownership in low and middle income countries could bring about a near doubling of road traffic deaths to 2.4 million per annum by 2030. A general growth in population numbers is likely to increase the number of deaths attributed to injuries by almost one-third by the year 2030. Non-communicable diseases will continue to grow in importance, with improvements in living standards and the availability of preventive health care.

Social inequalities in access to services

Most of us will require some care at the end of our lives, and the number of different agencies involved in caring for people at the end of their lives may be large. Appropriate care may incorporate any or all of mainstream health services, social services, charitable providers, private nursing homes, and family carers. The complexity of possible models of care on offer has grown in recent years, and this complexity also increases the likelihood that the quality and quantity of care will vary from place to place, and person to person. Thus, health care at the end of life is an area where the concept of equity may be very difficult to translate into practice. Nevertheless, the provision of equitable services, available according to need, and not ability to pay, age, ethnicity or any other characteristics, is an important goal for health systems. The measurement of access is not straightforward and utilization of care is often employed as a convenient proxy. It is far easier to measure who, or how many people used a health service, than it is to know who *could* have used it. Similarly, it is difficult to quantify the benefits that may accrue when a person knows that a service is available to them, even if they do not choose to use it. Differing educational levels, cultural and social experiences will mean that equal access will not necessarily lead to equal utilization. Use of services can be seen as a consequence of decisions, that are influenced by social context, the availability of services and the perception of the seriousness of the complaint. Some factors, such as age, family size, or ethnicity may predispose towards service use. Material resources— a car to go to hospital—or availability of a local service, would be important enabling factors (Andersen, 1995).

These are general limitations of research into access to health care, but they may be particularly important in end of life care, when a person's emotional and psychological well-being is so important. The knowledge that a community nurse is a telephone call away may make the difference between coping at home and admission to institutional care, for example. It follows that any analysis of a service should encompass affordability, geographical accessibility, and acceptability of services, not simply an adequate supply. It is also implicit that services are effective and appropriate, if they are to influence health outcomes.

End of life care for most people is provided by generalist health and social services; family doctors, community nurses and social carers. Specialist palliative care services see a relatively small proportion of all decedents in the UK, and a majority of their patients have a cancer diagnosis. In 2008–9 46,500 people were newly admitted for specialist inpatient care, representing fewer than 1 in 10 decedents. In the same year, around 113,000 new patients received specialist palliative home care (NCPC, 2010). Ensuring that access to primary and general medical care is fair, is clearly an essential part of delivering equitable end of life care. And for people with non-cancer diagnoses, with less predictable prognoses, good chronic disease management should be indistinguishable from end of life care.

In many health systems, the primary care doctor is both a provider of care and the gatekeeper to more specialist services. In countries with such a gatekeeper, access to primary care is generally found in studies to be equitable across the population, or, in many cases favours poorer people. Referral to secondary care is an important outcome of consultation with primary care practitioners and studies have shown that poor people tend to have lower rates of routine referral to specialist care, but higher rates of emergency hospitalizations (Hanratty et al., 2007a). In a study of hospital admissions within one English health authority area, deprivation at the GP practice level was positively correlated with emergency, but not routine admissions, a pattern that is repeated across other high-income countries such as Canada, the USA, and Finland. There are multiple possible causes for these differences, and it is unlikely that one single factor is responsible.

Financial barriers to end of life care

Financial stresses and strains at the end of life are well documented, and almost certain to have greater impact on low-income households (Hanratty et al., 2007b). Financial barriers to basic health care have been overcome to varying extents in high-income countries. Although around one in six of the population is without health insurance in the USA, people over 65 years, who make up the majority of decedents, and those on low incomes, have health care provided by federal and state funded safety net insurance schemes. In countries with universal coverage, health care is free at the point of access, but patients may face charges such as co-payments for medications, for example. For many families, rather than the costs of health care, it is the lost income associated with caring for family members, or the increased costs of living associated with the illness that have a greater effect on their household budgets. Travel to hospital, specific equipment or diets or increased heating may all be costly, when someone is ill at home. In qualitative research, these costs have been shown to be a greater burden at the end of life for lower income households (Hanratty, 2011).

Socio-economic barriers to access

It is many years since Tudor Hart (1971), then a family doctor in Wales, argued that the availability of good medical care tends to vary inversely with the need for the population served. Levels of morbidity and premature mortality are higher in poor areas, whereas doctors prefer to practise in more affluent urban areas. Tudor Hart was concerned with the malign influence of market forces when he described the inverse care law, and government intervention, either in the form of regulation of where doctors may practice (in the UK), or provision of safety net services (USA), is often used to ensure that a certain level of services is available to all. The geographical distribution of services also owes much to the historical origins of a service. In the UK, charitable organizations were behind the establishment of specialist palliative care, allowing the rapid development of services in the second half of the twentieth century. With the freedom to innovate, unconstrained by having to provide for all, they were able to create exemplary or special services where there was a drive to do so. By the 1980s, the service was described as inequitable, and concentrated in the affluent south-east of England (Lunt, 1985). Services are now available all across the UK, albeit with a wide inter-regional variation in the number of beds available.

Despite a widely held perception that hospice care was run by and for people in higher social groups, there is relatively little published evidence of socio-economic inequalities in access to specialist palliative care. Many of the relevant studies are of small scale, and Cartwright's study in the 1970s was the first large scale work to consider the issue (Cartwright, 1973). Interviews with almost 1,000 bereaved family carers across Britain explored the ways in which needs for medical, nursing and personal care were met. Although it produced valuable new insights into the plight of the dying, this study detected relatively few social class differences. People identified as working class relied more on children to supply care in their homes, whereas the middle classes on friends and neighbours, and there were some differences in place of death. In the follow-up study, more affluent people had a better quality of life and less financial hardship before death, even though they died at older ages.

Research using methods ranging from retrospective note review to qualitative interviews has failed to identify associations between social position and access to specialist palliative care for UK cancer patients (Kessler et al., 2005). Findings from other, robust studies are suggestive of inequities; less access to home care services for people in lower income groups, for example (Grande et al., 1998). Absence of evidence is always difficult to interpret, and there are reasons to remain sceptical about social patterns in service use. Place of death has attracted far greater interest from researchers than access to services, though the relationship with access to services is not necessarily straightforward. Secondly, the UK has one of the best established palliative care services in the world, and the situation is likely to be different in countries with fewer specialist services available. In Australia, a large state-wide survey found that uptake of specialist palliative care was lower in people with lower incomes and those whose first language was not English (Currow, 2008). Access to hospice care in the USA has been shown to vary with the proportion of graduates resident in the state. In contrast, age has consistently been found to be a barrier to access to specialist palliative care, for people with cancer and other diagnoses (Burt and Raine, 2006; Ahmed et al., 2004).

Delayed presentation

Equitable access to prompt treatment is an important goal in its own right, but it may also contribute to reducing social variation in the consequences of life limiting illnesses. Earlier diagnosis offers more opportunities to intervene in the course of an illness, and it may even change the outcome for an individual patient. The reasons why some people obtain medical help earlier than others have attracted a great deal of attention, particularly for conditions with a predictable disease trajectory, such as cancer. If the disease is more advanced at diagnosis, options for treatment may be fewer, quality of life worse, and survival shortened.

The social pattern in incidence of different diseases has led to suggestions that socio-economic status, and particularly educational attainment, may be a key factor explaining why some people do not receive treatment as soon as others. Delays may occur because patients fail to recognize the seriousness of their symptoms, or because they are frightened of what the symptoms may represent. Diagnosis may also be slow, if the health professional does not act promptly and order appropriate tests or make a timely referral when a patient consults them. Delay in seeking help for symptoms is common to a number of conditions including ischaemic heart disease, HIV, respiratory disease, and myocardial infarctions. A recent overview of research into the timing of cancer diagnoses suggests that the relationship between socio-economic status, educational attainment, and time to diagnosis and treatment varies with cancer site. People in lower socio-economic groups waited longer before their first consultations for symptoms of upper gastrointestinal and prostate cancer, but were sent more promptly for investigations for both upper GI and bowel cancers. Whereas education appeared to be the important factor in time to referral for gynaecological cancers (MacLeod et al., 2009).

Uptake of cancer screening is known to be greater amongst people in higher socio-economic groups, which may explain some of the variation in time to presentation of symptoms. This has been the case over decades of breast and cervical screening in the UK, and is illustrated by the ratio of screen detected to symptomatic breast cancers, where a relatively smaller proportion of breast cancers amongst poorer women were screen detected. Prostate and bowel screening programmes are relatively recent developments, but lower uptake of the screening blood test for prostate cancer and higher death rates have been reported in lower socio-economic groups in Switzerland, for example.

Place of death

As patient and family wishes have taken on a more prominent role in health policy and practice, the place where people are cared for at the end of their lives has assumed greater importance as an expression of patient autonomy and choice. Place of death has long been considered a proxy measure of good terminal care. More recently, it has been adopted as a process measure in the UK End of Life Strategy (Department of Health, 2008). The influences on where someone dies are wide-ranging and will inevitably vary with individual characteristics and prevailing social and cultural norms.

There are many other influences on the choices that people make about their care. Family carers' ability to cope mentally and physically with a burden of increasing care is usually central to any decisions made, whilst financial standing may be crucial in determining where someone receives their end of life care. Being able to afford care home fees can enable early admission, whereas an ability to purchase support, such as nursing care or equipment may all enable a person to stay at home, if that is their choice. With such wide-ranging influences, it is not surprising that research into associations between place of death and socio-economic status have produced conflicting results.

There is some evidence to support the hypothesis that higher socio-economic status is associated with greater likelihood and possibly preference for home death. In the UK, routine data show that a slightly higher proportion of people in the most deprived fifth of the population die in hospital (62% versus 55% in the least deprived quintile), or at home (20% versus 19%) (Ruth et al., 2010). Studies in countries ranging from Belgium and Canada to Korea have found that people living in more affluent neighbourhoods, or with higher educational qualifications, are more likely to die at home. However, the effect of socio-economic status is often modest, and in the US, the influence of racial and ethnic status may be difficult to disentangle from income inequalities in health or access to services. One nationally representative US study described racial and ethnic differences in place of death that could not be explained by income, age, or cause of death. Whereas other authors found a higher hospital death rate amongst non-white older Californians, and attributed much of the variation to lower socio-economic status amongst black and minority ethnic decedents.

A recent review of cancer deaths reported that six high-quality studies found an association with home death and social characteristics, such as higher education, income or social class. Although these studies were concerned with over 1.3 million people with cancer in the UK, Italy, Australia, and the USA, there were other studies that failed to find any association (Gomes and Higginson, 2006).

The area in which an individual lives, resources available, community and socio-cultural norms of behaviour are all powerful influences on health and health care utilization. Disadvantaged areas tend to be less well served by health and social care, and the availability of beds in hospitals or other institutions, and supportive care in the community has a strong association with place of death. In Spain, researchers have highlighted the importance of hospital provision, whereas in Belgium the availability of nursing homes has been identified as a strong influence on place of death.

Rural areas face related problems; services are naturally aligned with centres of population, and agricultural areas are generally low wage economies. Despite this, a high proportion of residents of rural areas have a home death. In sparsely populated areas, such as southern Australia, rural–urban differences in the use of hospice services are closely associated with place of death (Hunt et al., 2001). Similarly, in Taiwan, the home death rate is inversely related to the degree of urbanization. In these cases, distance from hospital or hospice facilities, and lower rates of car ownership amongst poorer communities may contribute to higher planned home deaths. It is also possible that some deaths at home are sudden. Premature cardiac deaths are more likely, for example, when the person with ischaemic heart disease is unable to reach medical care promptly.

The policy context

Services for people who are dying are influenced by general health and welfare policies, as well as by specific strategies that aim to improve the distribution and quality of care, such as the UK End of life Care Strategy. Health systems exist to care for patients, but they operate with constraints; containing costs, enhancing efficiency and for most, maintaining a certain level of equitable services. Inevitably, there will be overlap and sometimes conflict between policies that have a broader aim and the development needs of individual services. As population structures change, and the number of older people grows relative to economically active adults, concerns over funding have become one of the most important drivers of change in health care. This is pertinent to care at the end of life, as the majority of deaths in high-income countries are amongst the over-75s, an age group that is expected to double in size in European countries over the next 50 years. The months and years before death are often when service utilization and costs reach a lifetime high, making end of life care a significant component of the welfare bill.

Enhancing patient choice, moving care into community, and shifting responsibility from state to families and are common themes in health and social care policy across many high-income countries. Care at home is generally less costly than institutional care and preferred by patients and families, even though it will tend to increase the burden on both carers and community services. In disadvantaged areas, in particular, many family carers for older people are contributing many hours of unpaid care, despite being of advanced age themselves (Hanratty et al., 2007c). The UK health service has undergone quasi-market reforms in the last decade, allowing a diversity of providers within the NHS and giving patients greater choice of hospital. Hospitals were able to apply for greater financial and managerial freedom alongside more local accountability (Foundation Trust status). Changes were also made to the way in which hospitals were reimbursed for their services, with fixed tariff payments for activity replacing block contracts.

The introduction of greater choice of hospital provider may have limited impact on equity of access to health care, if the factors that allow a patient to exercise that choice are unaffected. Material resources, health beliefs and past experiences are likely to be influential, and vary with social position. To make a real difference to poorer patients, attention would need to be paid to the costs of accessing care, including time off work for family caregivers. Research to date has suggested that people value being offered some choice, but tend to continue to prefer their local provider (Dixon et al., 2010). At no time is this more likely to be the case than at the end of life, when timely, good quality local care would be preferred to more distant services. Many of the innovations that encourage plurality of providers and aim to improve value for money, introduce significant potential financial insecurity for providers and commissioners. If local services disappear as a result, it is the older, sicker, more disadvantaged patients who would be less able to travel distances for their care. A similar threat may be posed by the shift of service commissioning away from geographically defined populations to patients registered with groups of family doctors, proposed in the white paper, *Equity and Excellence: Liberating the NHS* (Department of Health, 2010).

The notion of choice has also been extended to purchasing services, with the personal budget schemes. They have been introduced in various forms in a number of countries around the world for social care, and in the UK, they are also being considered for health care. Although the schemes vary in structure, target groups and funding sources, they share common aims to contain costs, increase choice and autonomy for the users, and shift care into the community. In the UK, people eligible for social care have had the option of taking a direct payment from social services to fund their care since the mid-1990s. More recently, personalized budgets drawing on a number of public funding streams, have been introduced in pilot form in 13 local authorities in England. The local authority retains responsibility to ensure support is available, but the funds may be taken by the individual as a cash payment, or paid through a third party or care manager. The money can be used to purchase care from social services, voluntary organizations, the private sector or friends and family. Help and advice with planning a package of support may come from social workers, care managers, independent agencies or family. The introduction of cash payments in long-term care settings has been credited with stimulating competition in social care markets in Germany, France the Netherlands, and Sweden. Although the ability to purchase care is thought to be empowering, the underlying aim of the funding was to encourage family networks to provide care. Evaluation of the UK pilot project has found that older adults, the group most likely to be dealing with life limiting illnesses, saw the budget as an additional burden, and had greater levels of anxiety than other budget holders. It seems that older people will benefit from individualized budgets only if they are accompanied by substantial support and guidance (Glendinning et al., 2008). Eight areas in England are now introducing direct payments for aspects of health care, including, in one case, end of life care. This pilot scheme should be scrutinized carefully to ensure that families' need for support are being recognized.

Equitable financing

Fair financing of health services is an essential building block for equitable health care. It should go hand in hand with systematic assessment of population needs and rational planning of services. In the UK, the formulae devised to allocate funds between regions of the country provide an example of good practice, as they have attempted to account for the factors that may increase need and costs. These include material deprivation, age, ethnic make-up, and rurality, as well as supply side factors. Identifying how much money is spent on care for people who are dying, or elderly, or share the same diagnosis, is an inexact science. Few budgets are ring fenced at local level, and the complexity of end of life services, discussed previously, means that estimating costs for anything other than a specific service is a challenge. Linked administrative data-sets in Scandinavia permit analyses of resource utilization at individual level. A study from Stockholm showed that spending on health care in the last year of life decreases with age, over 65 years, but increases with socio-economic status, adjusting for age, sex, and diagnosis (Hanratty et al., 2007d). Data used for calculating charges in the USA permit similar analyses.

Financial incentives

The evidence that financial incentives for health providers can reduce inequalities in health or inequities in access to care, is limited. To date, most of the published research is from the UK, and concerned with primary care (Alshamsan et al., 2010). Payments for UK family doctors were linked to various activities in the new General Practitioner contract of 2003, to improve the quality and consistency of chronic disease management. Although almost all the UK studies described quality of care that was lower in disadvantaged compared to affluent areas, the size of the differences were small, and most disappeared in the early years of the incentive scheme. Differences by ethnicity, age, and sex persisted. There are fewer studies from the USA, where a wider range of incentives are found, reflecting the absence of a unified health system.

Financial incentives are available in UK general practice for aspects of end of life care. To qualify for the payments, GP practices must create a register of patients in need of palliative care, and discuss their condition at three-monthly multi-disciplinary meetings. This approach has been criticized for focusing on the process of care, as there is currently no requirement to demonstrate improved outcomes for patients on the palliative care register. The incentive aims to encourage consistent, high-quality care, and foster interdisciplinary communication. Patients who are entered into the register, may then gain privileged access to primary care services, with doctors more likely to visit at home, for example—which may be appropriate, good practice. But it also has the potential to create an elite group. People with cancer are certainly more likely to have their palliative care needs acknowledged. Ongoing evaluation will be crucial to ensure that this aspect of end of life care remains equitable, with the needs of patients and families determining access to services.

Care pathways and guidelines

Systematic approaches to end of life care have been introduced in a number of health systems. In the UK, the Gold Standards Framework and Liverpool Care Pathway have been widely adopted within the NHS. Their effect on social differences in the experience of dying has yet to be determined. To date, there is little evaluative evidence that care pathways are even effective (Chan and Webster, 2010), though this may reflect the specific outcome measures used in some reviews.

Conclusions

Our understanding and knowledge of social differences in morbidity and mortality is extensive. Our awareness of inequities in access to end of life services is fair. But our insight into how to address any inequalities is at a much earlier stage. Much of this chapter focused on the UK, where specialist palliative care has developed over decades, and health care is available to all, free at the point of access. It is reassuring that there is little evidence of extensive social differences in access to care in the UK, though the body of research is modest. If universal coverage is at the heart of the relative success of end of life care, proposed changes to the NHS may herald the end of a long period of development. Quasi market reforms, and the introduction of private providers introduce a new priority to health care, and the concern that profit may come before patients. Many innovations are untested. The ability of financial incentives to improve the quality and equity of end of life care in general practice is not yet proved, yet the scope of the project is being extended. Processes of care have changed, but the long-term impact on outcomes that are prized by the patients, remains to be seen. The challenge for the future is to ensure that every one of the 'million lights' described by Kubler-Ross receives the best care available at the end of their lives, wherever they live, and whatever their age, ethnic group, or medical condition. Achieving this must lie in critical scrutiny of existing service models combined with a determination to adhere to the values and principles articulated by Kubler-Ross and the other pioneers of end of life care.

Resources

- *Health Statistics Quarterly*, on the website of the Office for National Statistics in the UK, provides useful analyses of socio-economic trends in mortality in England and Wales: www.statistics.gov.uk/hub/health-social-care/index.html.
- For international data and analyses on health and health care, see the World Health Organization website: www.who.int/en/.
- The King's Fund is a charity that analyses health policy and conducts research relevant to the UK NHS. Its website contains a number of publications and reports relevant to equity and end of life care in England. See www.kingsfund.org.uk/.

References

Ahmed, N., Bestall, J. C., Ahmedzai, S. H., Payne, S. A., Clark, D., and Noble, B. (2004). Systematic review of the problems and issues of accessing specialist palliative care by patients, carers and health and social care professionals. *Palliative Medicine*, **18**: 525–42.

Alshamsan, R., Majeed, A., Ashworth, M., Car, J., and Millett, C. (2010). Impact of pay for performance on inequalities in health care: Systematic review. *Journal of Health Services & Research Policy*, **15**: 178–84.

Andersen, R. (1995). Revisiting the behavioral model and access to medical care: Does it matter? *Journal of Health and Social Behavior*, **36**: 1–10.

Burt, J. and Raine, R. (2006). The effect of age on referral to and use of specialist palliative care services in adult cancer patients: A systematic review. *Age & Ageing*, **35**: 469–76.

Cartwright, A., Hockely, L., and Anderson, J. L. (1973). *Life Before Death*. London: Routledge and Kegan Paul.

Chan, R. and Webster, J. (2010). End-of-life care pathways for improving outcomes in caring for the dying. *Cochrane Database of Systematic Reviews*, CD008006.

Currow, D. C., Agar, M., Sanderson, C., and Abernethy, A. P. (2008). Populations who die without specialist palliative care: Does lower uptake equate with unmet need? *Palliative Medicine*, **22**: 43–50.

Department of Health. (2008). *End of Life Care Strategy: Promoting High Quality Care for all Adults at the End of Life*. London: Stationary Office.

Department of Health. (2010). *Equity and Excellence: Liberating the NHS*. London: Stationary Office.

Dixon, A., Robertson, R., Appleby, J., Burge, P., Devlin, N., and Magee, H. (2010). *Patient Choice: How Patients Choose and How Providers Respond*. London: The King's Fund.

Faggiano, F., Partanen, T., Kogevinas, M., and Boffetta, P. (1997). Socioeconomic Differences in Cancer Incidence and Mortality. IARC Scientific Publications, **138**: 65–176.

Glendinning, C., Challis, D., Fernandez, J., Jacobs, S., Jones, K., et al. (2008). *Evaluation of the Individual Budgets Pilot Programme: Final Report*. York: Social Policy Research Unit, University of York.

Gomes, B. and Higginson, I. J. (2006). Factors influencing death at home in terminally ill patients with cancer: Systematic review. *BMJ*, **332**: 515–21.

Grande, G. E., Addington-Hall, J. M., and Todd, C. J. (1998). Place of death and access to home care services: Are certain patient groups at a disadvantage? *Social Science & Medicine*, **47**: 565–79.

Hanratty, B. (2011). Costs of Caring. In C. Ingleton and M. Gott (eds), *Living with Ageing and Dying*. Oxford: Oxford University Press.

Hanratty, B., Burstrom, B., Walander, A., and Whitehead, M. (2007d). Inequality in the face of death? Public expenditure on health care for different socioeconomic groups in the last year of life. *Journal of Health Services & Research Policy*, **12**: 90–4.

Hanratty, B., Drever, F., Jacoby, A., and Whitehead, M. (2007c). Retirement age caregivers and deprivation of area of residence. *European Journal of Ageing*, **4**: 35–43.

Hanratty, B., Holland, P., Jacoby, A., and Whitehead, M. (2007b). Financial stress and strain associated with terminal cancer—A review of the evidence. *Palliative Medicine*, **21**: 595–607.

Hanratty, B., Zhang, T., and Whitehead, M. (2007a). How close have universal health systems come to achieving equity in use of curative services? A systematic review. *International Journal of Health Services*, **37**: 89–109.

Hunt, R. W., Fazekas, B. S., Luke, C. G., and Roder, D. M. (2001). Where patients with cancer die in South Australia, 1990–1999: A population-based review. *Medical Journal of Australia*, **175**: 526–9.

Kessler, D., Peters, T. J., Lee, L., and Parr, S. (2005). Social class and access to specialist palliative care services. *Palliative Medicine*, **19**: 105–10.

Lunt, B. (1985). Terminal cancer care services: Recent changes in regional inequalities in Great Britain. *Social Science & Medicine*, **20**: 753–9.

Macleod, U., Mitchell, E. D., Burgess, C., Macdonald, S., and Ramirez, A. J. (2009). Risk factors for delayed presentation and referral of symptomatic cancer: Evidence for common cancers. *British Journal of Cancer*, **101**(Suppl. 2): S92–S101.

National Council for Palliative Care. (2010). *National Survey of Patient Activity Data for Specialist Palliative Care Services: MDS Full Report 2008/09*. London: The National Council for Palliative Care.

Office for National Statistics. (2010). *Health Inequalities in the 21st Century*, www.statistics.gov.uk/statbase/Product.asp?vlnk=15056 . Accessed 22 Nov. 2010.

Riley, J. C. (2001). *Rising Life Expectancy: A Global History*. Cambridge: Cambridge University Press.

Ruth, K., Pring, A., and Verne, J. (2010). Variations in place of death in England: Inequalities or appropriate consequences of age, gender and cause of death. South West Public Health Observatory (www.swpho.nhs.uk).

Strand, B. H., Kunst, A., Huisman, M., Menvielle, G., Glickman, M., Bopp, M., et al. and the EU Working Group on Socioeconomic Inequalities in Health. (2007). The reversed social gradient: Higher breast cancer mortality in the higher educated compared to lower educated. A comparison of 11 European populations during the 1990s. *European Journal of Cancer*, **43**: 1200–7.

Tudor Hart, J. (1971). The Inverse Care Law. *Lancet*, **1**: 405–12.

United Nations. (2010). Population and Vital Statistics Report. Statistical Papers Series A. New York: Department of Economic and Social Affairs, United Nations.

Chapter 4

Place and space: Geographic perspectives on death and dying

Anthony C. Gatrell and Sheila Payne

Introduction

There cannot be very many published papers, or contributions to edited collections, that combine the perspective of a geographer—long interested in how place and space relate to health and well-being—and the perspective of a psychologist (with a background in nursing) whose academic research embraces problems concerning care, and care provision, for those at or nearing the end of their lives. We seek to combine our disciplinary strengths in order to reveal how a geographical imagination can serve to illuminate some of the most pressing concerns of late-modern society; the needs of those facing death. Such needs will embrace, in particular, the settings where people die and the differential 'access' to, and quality of, such settings.

It may help, at the outset, to illustrate such a geographical imagination with three key questions that inform debates on death and dying.

Q1: To what extent is place of death shaped by geographical proximity to sites of provision such as specialist in-patient hospices?

Q2: Are there inequalities in the geographical location of palliative care services, with some areas 'under-served' compared with others and, if so, are the under-served areas characterized by relative socio-economic deprivation?

Q3: While issues of geographical accessibility to sites of care are important, what are the restorative or therapeutic environmental qualities of such places for people who use them or work in them?

Approaches to answering each of these sorts of questions are described in this chapter.

Before we address these important issues we need to set our chapter in context. In particular, we introduce readers to what we understand by a 'geographical imagination' (perhaps, more accurately, 'imaginations') and how these speak to those interested in health, well-being, and health care delivery. We therefore look briefly at what is meant by 'medical geography' and how, over the past 20 years, disciplinary perspectives have shifted from descriptions and analyses of patterns of mortality (and morbidity) to those which bring the social and cultural into play, informing what is now called 'health geography' (Gatrell and Elliott, 2009).

In the second main section we shall use this context to review some of the literature on geographies of death and dying, with a particular focus on 'place of death'. Here, we consider the rich and growing body of literature that looks at the geography of place of death. We review those studies, essentially quantitative in orientation, of variation in place of death. We subsequently contrast those with other studies that look in more detail, and in more nuanced ways, at the settings, or places themselves. In other words, the focus shifts from the study of multiple places (treated as rather abstract locations) towards an examination of the settings as places imbued with meaning for those who encounter them as sites of care.

In the third section we again contrast two broad approaches. We first look at quantitative approaches to planning the location of care services and how relatively modern methods (such as Geographic Information Systems) can be used to assess the accessibility to, and use of, services provided for those nearing the end of life. But we contrast those with studies which examine the experience of care and what are now called 'emotional geographies'.

Medical and health geography

The sub-discipline of medical geography has a long and distinguished history, with a dual focus on, first, mapping, describing and seeking to explain the geographic or spatial distribution of disease (both mortality and morbidity) and, second, on examining locational patterns of health care delivery and use. Each is considered briefly.

The first area of study is concerned with static pictures of disease prevalence or incidence. So, for example, we could map the spatial distribution of cancer mortality in a country or region, with particular sub-regions (counties, electoral districts perhaps) as the units of analysis. Classically, this form of spatial epidemiology would look for patterns in the map (and there are many techniques for doing just that: see Pfeiffer et al., 2008, for a fine overview) but would go beyond simple description to try to explain the distribution, using environmental or socio-economic data, as appropriate.

To make this more concrete consider the work undertaken in the US by the National Cancer Institute (NCI): http://cancercontrolplanet.cancer.gov/atlas/index.jsp. This allows one to produce customizable maps, by state, by county, and by State Economic Area, for 37 cancer sites, and by age, gender, 'race', and time period. As a means of visualizing and exploring mortality due to cancer the results are compelling. For example, high rates of lung cancer in the 'deep south' are shown clearly, while the converse is true for colo-rectal cancers; higher death rates in some of the so-called 'rust belt' areas of the north-east. For Britain, Shaw and her colleagues (2008) have produced a mortality atlas by parliamentary constituency (voting area) over the period 1981–2004. This includes over 14 million deaths, by 99 causes, converted into standardized mortality ratios. Results are presented as cartograms—maps in which geographical areas are replaced by (in this case) hexagonal cells that are coloured according to mortality ratio. This is a common cartographic device; see similar unconventional maps for all countries: www.worldmapper.org/. It is, of course, entirely descriptive in nature but can be used to frame hypotheses of causation. Consequently, data on other variables can be collected that potentially explain the spatial distributions and there is a huge literature on this, looking at spatial variation in particular countries. There are very sophisticated methods employed here, that take into account the fact that the observations in spatial units are not independent (as in classical statistical analysis) but are correlated. For example, Borrell et al. (2010) have modelled spatial variation in mortality (for all causes and selected causes of death, between 1996 and 2003) in census tracts for 11 Spanish cities. Their results show that levels of socio-economic deprivation within small areas explain substantial proportions of variation in mortality.

This Spanish study is illustrative of the considerable interest, over the last 15 years, in the impact of income inequality on ill-health, but also on mortality, research triggered in part by Wilkinson's (1996) book (but recently updated in Wilkinson and Pickett, 2009). The argument, briefly, is that those advanced industrial countries (or regions) in which incomes are more evenly distributed have better health outcomes (or lower mortality) than those with higher levels of income inequality. Studies in the USA (for example, Kennedy et al., 1996) reveal that while mortality is only weakly associated with average income by state, it is correlated significantly with income distribution.

While useful, in this kind of study the results can be affected by the scale of analysis (for example, different results can be obtained, depending on whether analysis is conducted at the state or county level in the USA) and by the fact that the units themselves are somewhat arbitrary (in other words, if the boundaries were drawn differently the results would change). Where possible therefore, some researchers prefer to analyse data on individuals. However, methods such as multi-level modelling (Gould, 2010) can be used that link aggregate and individual analysis. For example, if we had individual death records and ancillary data for such individuals we could model mortality as both a function of risk factors pertaining to individuals (smoking history, perhaps) and contextual variables relating to environmental quality in, and socio-economic characteristics of, the local neighbourhood.

To illustrate this, consider two studies. Jerrett and his colleagues (2010) report on a study of mortality in Los Angeles that uses multi-level modelling to examine the impact of air pollution on various causes of death (including ischaemic heart disease). Controlling for individual influences they find significant associations between particulate air pollution (including that from vehicle exhaust emissions) and mortality. Second, Dahl and colleagues (2006) have explored regional variations in mortality in Norway, with a particular interest in assessing whether levels of income inequality in 88 regions had any impact on mortality during the 1990s, over and above individual determinants (such as age, sex, family income, and education). Using data for over 2 million individuals their results suggested that, among those with low individual income, low education, and recipients of welfare benefits, the effects of higher levels of regional income inequality on mortality were significantly greater than for those more advantageously placed in the social structure. This suggests that 'context' matters; specifically, despite Norway having a relatively equal distribution of income and a fair welfare system there were nonetheless regional-level income inequality effects on mortality, these effects being particularly marked among socio-economically disadvantaged groups.

In most of these (spatial) analyses, space is simply seen as a container for data on health outcomes and potential explanatory variables. The areal units of analysis are rather abstract, divorced of any social meaning. As we see shortly, there are other approaches to understanding death in a spatial context.

In the second broad area of application geographers have sought to determine the optimal locations of public sector facilities (such as hospitals or health centres) as well as their accessibility to the populations that might wish to use them (see Tanser et al., 2010, for an overview). Those people who live relatively close to health facilities are more likely to use them and reap the benefits of so doing. Such methods require data on the locations of centres of care, as well as data on the geographical distribution of the population that might need to use them. They also require data on the distance between centres of supply and demand; at its most simple such data might be straight line distances, but more sophisticated approaches use estimated journey times by road. Regardless, the methods used in this kind of study tend to look exclusively at the locations of service centres, and rarely concern themselves with service characteristics or service quality. Rather, they seek to describe, and perhaps improve, locational distributions in order to optimize accessibility. This is an entirely laudable goal, though the implication of 'modern' rational planning has proved unappealing for some tastes. Further, such studies assume that health care is consumed within fixed-site institutions rather than by a model of 'outreach' where care is given at home or in other non-institutional settings. This is an important caveat, as we see later.

These classical concerns, whether with the distribution of mortality or of health facilities, began to give way, particularly during the 1990s, to approaches that focused less on location and more on 'place'; specifically, places as suffused with social meaning and cultural life. Researchers sought to bring people back into the frame, not as dots on maps or anonymous particles that could be aggregated into spatial units for the purpose of (quantitative) analysis but, rather, as knowledgeable actors with feelings, beliefs, and health experiences. In so doing the sub-discipline underwent a conversion from a medical model of health and disease, in which the focus was on describing and explaining the geographic distribution of diseased bodies, to an emphasis on health and well-being; put differently, a desire not merely to map death and illness but to understand why some bodies were sick, or in the process of becoming so. Researchers thereby began to draw on a range of social science perspectives (reviewed in Gatrell and Elliott, 2009). As for an interest in accessibility, interest shifted away from merely measuring levels of access, towards an understanding of the experience of particular health care settings; what were they *like* as sites of health care consumption?

In sum, while it is an over-simplification, we can think of a shift, in geographical studies, from a medicalized focus on *space*, to a health-related focus on textured *places*.

From geographies of mortality to place of death

Those approaching the geography of health from an overtly medical perspective have, as indicated above, contributed to a vast literature on geographical variation on mortality. But there is also now a substantial literature on 'place of death', including studies in a number of countries and a focus on the relationship between actual place of death and preferred place of death. In this literature 'place of death' usually refers to 'setting', and studies typically describe, and seek to explain, the proportions of deaths at home or in hospital, or in other settings such as nursing and care homes or hospices.

Curiously, geographers have rather neglected this as an area of study; indeed, they have, in the main, made relatively few contributions to the geographical dimensions of palliative care.

From a distinctively *geographical* perspective the question of interest in this section is whether there is spatial variation in the settings where people die, and what might account for such variation. In other words, does the probability of death at home (or in a hospital, or specialist in-patient hospice) death vary from country to country, from region to region, or more locally, and if so what factors might account for this? Such factors might include those relating to the individual (their age, sex, family circumstances, socio-economic status, or diagnosed condition) but might also include the kinds of contextual factors alluded to above.

At the global scale a recent report has drawn sharp contrasts between countries in terms of 'quality of death' (Economist Intelligence Unit, 2010). Using data on availability, cost and quality of end of life care, along with 'health care environment' the report positions the UK at the head of a 'league table', followed by Australia and New Zealand; Canada and the US are ranked equal 9th, with the so-called 'BRIC' countries (Brazil, Russia, India, and China) ranked 35th or lower. The lack of facilities, lack of opioids, and cultural attitudes to death (such as an unwillingness to accept that death is imminent) help to explain why some countries are ranked low. As Beccaro et al. (2007) argue, the world-wide development of palliative care teams (either domiciliary or hospital-based) and hospices reflects different health care systems, culture, and varying patient need. Within Europe, Rocafort and Centeno (2008) have reviewed, in a very comprehensive way, country-by-country variation in palliative care (covering, for example, types of provision, opioid availability, and education).

Some studies are fundamentally descriptive, seeking to outline geographical variations in place of death. For example, Mystakidou and colleagues (2009) looked at the changing relative proportions of home-based and hospital deaths from cancer in three regions of Greece. Nearly 60% of both men and women die in hospital, proportions that are higher in central Greece but slightly lower in Macedonia. An Italian study of provision and use of palliative care for cancer patients describes geographical variations but goes beyond these to explain differences in care (Beccaro et al., 2007). For example, in southern Italy almost one-half (48%) of patients were cared for exclusively at home, with 2.3% referred to domiciliary palliative care teams. Care in nursing homes and hospital were more common in the north, where about 18% of patients were referred to domiciliary palliative care teams. The involvement of pain specialists varied by region too. As the authors put it, there are 'clear geographical differences reflecting an unequal provision of and access to palliative care services across the country' (Beccaro et al., 2007).

In an important recent study in England the National End of Life Care Intelligence Network (NEoLCIN) has brought together a rich set of data on end of life care that can be mapped by Local Authority. It provides the facility to map data by age, gender, cause of death and—crucially for the present chapter—place of death. See: www.endoflifecare-intelligence.org.uk/profiles.aspx. As an example Figure 4.1 shows a 'screen grab' including a map of female deaths at home during 2005–7. Inspection of

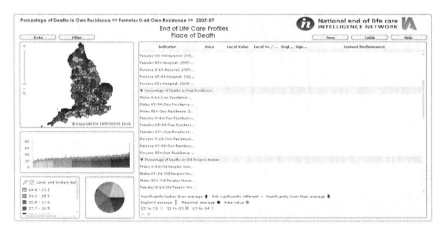

Fig. 4.1 Proportion of female deaths at home, 2005–7 (*source*: NEoLCIN, reproduced with permission).

the data using the interactive software reveals relatively high percentages of such deaths in rural areas. For example, almost two-thirds (64%) of such deaths in Berwick-on-Tweed (on the border with Scotland) are at home whereas in Dartford and Haringey in London the percentages are under 15%. To give another example, data on the percentage of deaths in hospices, in which cancer is given as the underlying cause of death, reveals that Milton Keynes 'tops the league' (12% of such deaths) while the percentage is only 0.1% in rural Copeland in Cumbria. This comprehensive set of data (soon to be updated with 2007–9 mortality data: NEoLCIN, personal communication, 20 September 2010) will prove invaluable for further research and in policy-making.

Other studies have looked at much more local geographical variation. Of interest to the writers has been the geographical availability of particular health care settings within the UK. For example, the probability of a hospice death depends on there being available a hospice within a 'reasonable' distance of one's home. In part of north-west England the presence of two hospices meant that a relatively high proportion of deaths (33%) were in that setting, and 35% in hospital (Gatrell et al., 2003). Logistic regression modelling using data for almost 7,000 individual cancer deaths revealed that the probability of dying in a hospice was significantly higher among younger cancer patients and those with lymphatic cancer. Importantly, it was also related to proximity to hospice. The study used digital data on road networks to determine the travel distance from home to hospice. This illustrates the point that data on geographical availability of services are required in order to explain adequately the proportion of deaths in hospice (or at home): also see Higginson et al. (1999).

Wilson and her colleagues (2006) have reviewed studies of the provision of end of life care in rural areas in the developed world. Predictably, the tendency is for deaths of rural dwellers to be more common at home. Specialist palliative care services serving rural areas are relatively rare, and while rural community hospitals provide general palliative care (Payne et al., 2004) the majority of care is provided by family members because formal home nursing care is limited.

From health care planning to landscapes of care

Some palliative care services have been 'piecemeal, unplanned, and largely unregulated [thereby exacerbating] disparities in access to receiving care by geographic location and socio-economic status' (Cinnamon et al., 2008). But whether services have been developed (and located) in a planned way, or instead have emerged less systematically, there is a need to assess whether service provision is equitable; in other words, whether those in most need find that such services are 'accessible'. 'Access' is a term that has multiple meanings. In a geographical context it means whether services are located such that they can be reached in reasonable time. This is the primary concern in what follows.

There is a growing number of studies making use of Geographical Information Systems (GIS) to assess locational accessibility. A GIS is a computerized system for collecting, manipulating, mapping and analysing geographical data (see Gatrell and Elliott, 2009, Chapter 3). If we know the locations of palliative care services, have digital data on road networks (which allow us to estimate likely travel times) and data on population distribution, we can use GIS to define 'catchment areas' around particular facilities as well as highlighting areas that appear to be under-served. This is likely to prove particularly important for older populations—those more likely to be accessing palliative care services—who, along with potential carers, may be less mobile than other demographic groups.

Research groups in Canada and the UK have been active in exploring the uses of these methods in end of life care, particularly in the assessment of geographic access to specialist palliative care. Cinnamon and his colleagues (2008) digitized the locations of hospices and hospitals with designated palliative care units (with a minimum of five beds) in British Columbia. They then determined, for each of the 29 facilities, catchment areas that represented a maximum notional drive time of one hour. Within each catchment they used Census data to compute the total population that is potentially served by the facility. This revealed marked geographical disparities. For example, in the north of the province only 36% of the population was within one hour of a facility, while in the Vancouver city region about 90% of the population was served. This is an interesting exercise, though as the authors note it may, like other studies 'discount the efforts of informal caregivers and non-specialized types of care which also likely benefit the patient at the end of life' (Cinnamon et al., 2008). In other words, unless services have fixed geographic allocations, the methods are not appropriate. One might also criticize the study for assuming that total population is the appropriate measure of service 'demand'.

An earlier study involving one of the authors (Wood et al., 2004) took a slightly different approach. Set in north-west England, it sought to assess the extent to which those living in small localities (electoral wards, comprising populations of c.5,000 people) had equity of access to adult in-patient hospices. The study used estimated journey times between hospices and localities to determine geographical accessibility, but also incorporated simple data on 'supply' (hospice bed numbers), the argument being that proximity to a hospice with more beds was likely to be more attractive than to one with fewer bed spaces. Demand for hospice services was taken to be not simply total population but, rather, estimates of cancer incidence; this is quite reasonable

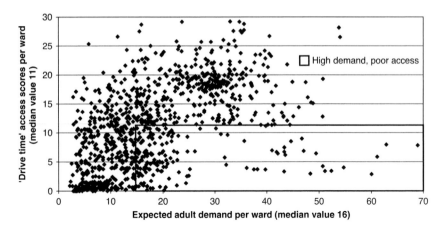

Fig. 4.2 Relationship between accessibility to adult in-patient hospice services and expected demand, by small area in north-west England (*source*: Wood et al., 2004).

given that well over 90% of referrals to in-patient hospices are of people with cancer (Coupland et al., 2010). A further innovation was to incorporate data on socio-economic deprivation. Consequently, as well as identifying small areas that were relatively remote from hospices the research was able to see which relatively inaccessible areas were also those that had high 'need'. Results are illustrated in Figures 4.2 and 4.3. In Figure 4.2 the relationship between an accessibility score ('supply') and cancer incidence ('demand') for each small area is depicted; the box indicates those small areas where access is below the median and cancer incidence is above the median. That subset of small areas can be mapped, though a further restriction to identify only those areas where deprivation is above average (Figure 4.3) is the main focus of interest. This suggests that there are some coastal locations that would benefit from additional provision. Of course, the study has limitations, some shared with the British Columbia work. It only examined in-patient hospice provision, and there are plenty of other forms of support (day care, home-based care, hospital support teams, and so on) that may provide care in the identified 'under-served' areas. Thus the supply side was treated somewhat simplistically. Equally, the demand side needs further refinement, since not all those with cancer require palliative care while hospices increasingly care for those with non-cancer diagnoses. Nonetheless, the research was instructive and illustrated the value of a geographical approach that used modern (GIS) analytical methods.

More recently, Wood (2010), working with the two writers and others, has extended this research to the whole of the UK, examining issues of accessibility but also the actual utilization of specialist in-patient hospices. Detailed findings will be reported soon in the literature but, briefly, his examination of the probability of dying in such hospices is shown to be significantly inversely related to geographical accessibility and significantly positively associated with socio-economic deprivation.

Members of the research group working in British Columbia have extended their earlier GIS approach to examine the importance of 'place' in a more nuanced way

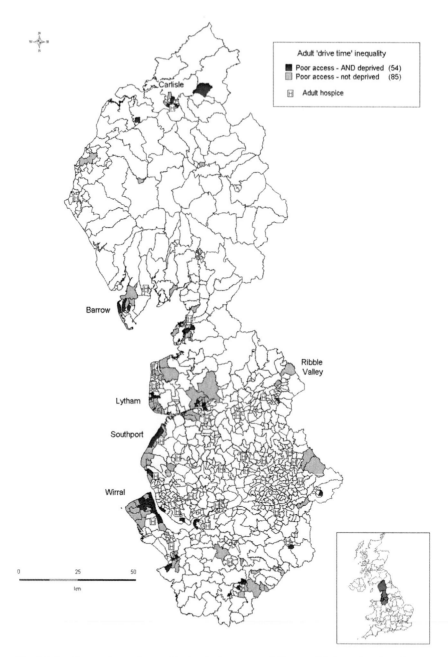

Fig. 4.3 Small areas in north-west England where accessibility to adult in-patient hospice services is below average and demand is above average, classified by socio-economic deprivation (*source*: Wood et al., 2004).

(Castleden et al., 2010). Rather than simply look at the physical distance separating home and fixed locations that deliver palliative care, they look at such locations, in rural parts of the province, more in terms of the aesthetics of such locations. Conversations with both providers and users revealed that the appearance of settings—the quality of the local environment, its internal architecture and decor, as well as the 'soundscape' and 'smellscape', were key components of the experience of palliative care. Relative location (proximity to care settings) was of course important, particularly given the low density of population and the dispersed care settings, as well as the difficulty of driving conditions in winter months. But settings are not simply fixed locations on a map; they are places infused with social meaning—whether family homes, the regional hospital or other care facilities. A good death is facilitated by spending time in aesthetically attractive places, with family and friends nearby. For many though, the attractions of rural living are seen differently as death approaches: 'the sense of *solitude* afforded to life in the rural idyll can become a sense of *isolation* for those who are approaching end of life ... and the *caring nature* of rural communities can be replaced with care providers having to negotiate a seemingly *compassionless system*' (Castleden et al., 2010: 288; their italics).

While geographers and epidemiologists have long argued that aspects of the physical environment (air and water quality, now climate change) can have major impacts on physical health outcomes it has been less frequently argued that the (physical and material) environment can help shape mental health and well-being, whether for those approaching their end of life of for others needing health care. A shift in focus from geographical access to the experiential qualities of care settings is illustrated in work done on gardens as places for contemplation, either for terminally ill patients in a hospice or hospital, or as places where carers and visitors can seek 'restorative respite from stressful caring demands' (Hartig and Cooper Marcus, 2006; see also an earlier paper by Healy, 1986). One reason why those nearing the end of life would prefer to die at home is doubtless because it is a familiar and comforting environment, made all the more so perhaps by views from the window.

This work relates to wider concerns in health geography with 'nature as nurture'— the engagement of people with attractive and appealing natural environments to which they can connect and derive emotional sustenance. Research on so-called 'therapeutic landscapes'—places associated with maintaining and promoting health—has been employed in the palliative care literature, particularly to assess the quality of care delivered in the home (Donovan and Williams, 2007). This connects with wider debates (see Milligan and Power, 2010, for a review) on the changing geography of health and social care. Such research is in part concerned with the spatial organization of the domestic setting (the physical arrangements of furniture and material resources) but more with shifting practices within the home. As Milligan and Power observe, the home becomes a site of both production (care work) and consumption, creating complex patterns of power relationships between those in receipt of care, and those giving care (including health and social care professionals and family members). What were once private spaces for family members get 'opened up' to others, changing the meaning of the home-place. Moreover, the care recipient, particularly at the end of life, is potentially very restricted in terms of her or his access to domestic space. And, as many authors have noted, the burden of care usually falls on women, with possible consequences for their own well-being and a sharpening of the 'social differences' (by gender) with which this book is concerned. While the home may be a therapeutic place for the care recipient, for the family care-giver there are costs, emotional and financial, that have to be borne (see Donovan and Williams, 2007, for empirical research on this in a Canadian context). Much depends on the material resources available; it may well be easier to re-organize the home-space in a large house than in a small city apartment, implying that those who are better-off have better 'access' to care than those who are materially disadvantaged. As with any setting—home, hospital or in-patient hospice— the environment can be health-enhancing as well as health-detracting.

Concluding remarks

As the contributions to this edited volume suggest, there are many dimensions to the inequalities in death and dying. Some of the evidence reviewed above suggests that these inequalities have a distinctly *spatial* dimension. In particular, if policy-makers are serious about increasing the provision of specialist in-patient hospices (as physical sites) they need to acknowledge that the locations of such sites can shape geographical accessibility. Usage of such facilities will be shaped by a variety of factors, but relative location is assuredly one of them.

Set alongside these traditional concerns with relative location, however, we must not neglect other important questions on the geography of death and dying. Again, if we are serious—as we surely must be—about enabling a 'good death', we have to recognize that care towards and at the end of life has to take place some*where* (despite moves by some to provide care in virtual environments), and we have to examine the qualities of those settings and the meanings that care recipients, carers, and health professionals attach to them. Location and place cannot be ignored as shapers of palliative care and of the experience of such care.

Resources

- ◆ See Gatrell and Elliott (2009) for an introduction to the geography of health, including discussions of methodological approaches, research methods, and areas of study (including health inequalities and service provision).
- ◆ For a geographical perspective on health inequalities see the collection edited by Boyle et al. (2004).
- ◆ For a comprehensive set of chapters that review all aspects of health geography see the collection edited by Brown et al. (2010).

References

Beccaro, M., Costantini, M., Merlo, D., and the ISDOC Study Group. (2007). Inequity in the provision of and access to palliative care for cancer patients. Results from the Italian survey of the dying of cancer (ISDOC), *BMC Public Health*, **7**: 66.

Borrell, C., Marí-Dell'olmo, M., Serral, G., Martínez-Beneito, M., Gotsens, M., and MEDEA Members. (2010). Inequalities in mortality in small areas of eleven Spanish cities (the multicenter MEDEA project). *Health & Place*, **16**: 703–11.

Boyle, P., Curtis, S., Graham, E., and Moore, E. (eds) (2004). *The Geography of Health Inequalities in the Developed World*. Aldershot, UK: Ashgate.

Brown, T., McLafferty, S., and Moon, G. (eds) (2010). *A Companion to Health and Medical Geography*. Oxford: Wiley-Blackwell.

Castleden, H., Crooks, V. A., Schuurman, N., and Hanlon, N. (2010). 'It's not necessarily the distance on the map . . . ': Using place as an analytic tool to elucidate geographic issues central to rural palliative care. *Health & Place*, **16**: 284–90.

Cinnamon, J., Schuurman, N., and Crooks, V. A. (2008). A method to determine spatial access to specialized palliative care services using GIS. *BMC Health Services Research*, **8**: 140.

Coupland, V. H., Lee, W., Madden, P., Sykes, N., Heal, R., Moller, H., and Davies, E. A. (2010). Is it possible to determine use of hospice palliative care services by matching hospice and cancer registry data? *Palliative Medicine*, **24**: 807–11.

Dahl, E., Ivar Elstad, J., Hofoss, D., and Martin-Mollard M. (2006). For whom is income inequality most harmful? A multi-level analysis of income inequality and mortality in Norway. *Social Science and Medicine*, **63**: 2562–74.

Donovan, R. and Williams, A. (2007). Home as therapeutic landscape: Family caregivers providing palliative care at home. In A. Williams (ed.), *Therapeutic Landscapes*. Aldershot, UK: Ashgate.

Economist Intelligence Unit. (2010). *The Quality of Death: Ranking End-of-life Care Across the World*. London: Economist Intelligence Unit.

Gatrell, A. C. and Elliott, S. J. (2009) *Geographies of Health*. Oxford: Wiley-Blackwell.

Gatrell, A. C., Harman, J. C., Francis, B. J., Thomas, C., Morris, S. M., and McIllmurray, M. (2003). Place of death: Analysis of cancer deaths in part of north-west England. *Journal of Public Health Medicine*, **25**: 53–8.

Gould, M. (2010). Modeling chronic disease. In T. Brown, S. McLafferty, and G. Moon (eds), *A Companion to Health and Medical Geography*. Oxford: Wiley-Blackwell.

Hartig, T. and Cooper Marcus, C. (2006). Healing gardens–Places for nature in health care, medicine and creativity. *The Lancet*, **368**: S36–7.

Healy, V. (1986). The hospice garden: Addressing the patient's needs through landscape. *American Journal of Hospice Care*, **3**: 18–23.

Higginson, I., Jarman, B., Astin, P., and Dolan, S. (1999). Do social factors affect where patients die: An analysis of 10 years of cancer deaths in England. *Journal of Public Health Medicine*, **21**: 22–8.

Jerrett, M., Gale, S., and Kontgis, C. (2010). An environmental health geography of risk. In T. Brown, S. McLafferty, and G. Moon (eds), *A Companion to Health and Medical Geography*. Oxford: Wiley-Blackwell.

Kennedy, B. P., Kawachi, I., and Prothrow-Stith, D. (1996). Income distribution and mortality: Cross-sectional ecological study of the Robin Hood index in the US. *British Medical Journal*, **312**: 1004–7.

Milligan, C. and Power, A. (2010). The changing geography of care. In T. Brown, S. McLafferty, and G. Moon (eds), *A Companion to Health and Medical Geography*. Oxford: Wiley-Blackwell.

Mystakidou, K., Tsilika, E., Galanos, A., and Theodorakis, P. (2009). The incidence of place of death in Greek patients with cancer in 1995 and 2005. *American Journal of Hospice & Palliative Medicine*, **26**: 347–53.

Payne, S., Kerr, C., Hawker, S., Seamark, D., Davis, C., Roberts, H., Jarrett, N., Roderick, P., and Smith, H. (2004). A Survey of the Provision of Palliative Care in Community Hospitals: An unrecognised resource. *Journal of the Royal Society of Medicine*, **97**: 428–31.

Pfeiffer, D., Robinson, T., Stevenson, M., Stevens, K., Rogers, D., and Clements, A. (2008). *Spatial Analysis in Epidemiology*. Oxford: Oxford University Press.

Rocafort, J. and Centeno, C. (2008). *EAPC Review of Palliative Care in Europe*. Milan: European Association for Palliative Care.

Shaw, M., Thomas, B., Davey Smith, G., and Dorling, D. (2008). *The Grim Reaper's Road Map: An Atlas of Mortality in Britain*. Bristol: The Policy Press.

Tanser, F., Gething, P., and Atkinson, P. (2010). Location-allocation planning. In T. Brown, S. McLafferty, and G. Moon (eds), *A Companion to Health and Medical Geography*. Oxford: Wiley-Blackwell.

Wilkinson, R. G. (1996). *Unhealthy Societies: The Afflictions of Inequality*. London: Routledge.

Wilkinson, R. G. and Pickett, K. (2009). *The Spirit Level: Why More Equal Societies Almost Always do Better*. London: Allen Lane.

Wilson, D. M., Justice, C., Sheps, S., Thomas, R., Reid, P., and Leibovici, K. (2006). Planning and providing end-of-life care in rural area, *Journal of Rural Health*, **22**: 174–81.

Wood, D. J. (2010). Equity of geographic access of specialist inpatient hospices within the United Kingdom. PhD thesis, Lancaster University.

Wood, D. J., Clark, D., and Gatrell, A. C. (2004). Equity of access to adult hospice inpatient care within north-west England. *Palliative Medicine*, **18**: 543–9.

Chapter 5

Communication, information, and support

May McCreaddie

'The problem with communication is the illusion that it has occurred.'

George Bernard Shaw

Introduction

'Communication' and 'information needs and support' have been contemporary
and contested issues in health care generally and end of life care in particular.
Communication (and information as part of that) is not something that simply gets
done—like taking a blood pressure or cardio-pulmonary resuscitation—and therefore, a 'task' that (only) requires a certain skill set to be acquired and applied. Rather,
as Duke (2010), in a recent guest editorial for the *European Journal of Oncology Nursing*
suggests, communication *per se* needs a much broader conceptualization; as a complex, mutable phenomenon at the mercy of interpersonal and contextual factors—a
process, not an outcome or an end-point. Certain aspects of communication such as
patients' *information needs* and health care staffs' *communication skills* are important
but they are only part of what is a dynamic, human(e) phenomenon.

What are the key issues and what do patients want?

The diagnosis of a terminal disease is patently a traumatic and challenging experience
for patients, their partners, families, and friends. Making sense of what is happening
and dealing with these challenges is, to a greater or lesser degree, dependent upon *what*
information and support is provided by *who, how, when, where,* and *to whom*. For
example, each patient will respond differently to any given situation across the care
trajectory from diagnosis through treatment decisions to end of life care. *Information
needs* will therefore vary accordingly. However, the majority of research on information
needs appears to focus on tangible issues such as diagnosis, treatment and therapies
(Adams et al., 2009). The more concrete, specific and individual aspects of illness such
as psychosocial issues, sexuality needs, continence or the legalities of writing a will and
the more challenging emotive aspects such as 'survivorship' or the transition from living
to dying are notably less prominent (Cappiello et al., 2007).

Information needs: a moral imperative?

Innumerable papers have attempted to unlock the door to information nirvana since Cassilleth et al. (1980) first highlighted the 'information needs' of patients. The notion that information should be provided and that most patients want and seek information (see Mayer et al., 2007) appears relatively uncontested. Accordingly, the pro-information lobby cite the potential for countless benefits including: increased involvement of the patient in decision-making, reduced anxiety increased ability to cope/psychological well-being, improved therapeutic relationships/patient satisfaction, increased communication with family members/relevant others—to name but a few.

Information-seeking, the purposeful acquisition of information, *presumes* that individuals desire information and, therefore, wish to participate in their care and decisions affecting their care. Indeed, the concept of a 'good death' is based upon an awareness of diagnosis and prognosis and the concomitant ability to participate in advance care planning. Providing information is apparently a good thing, a moral imperative. However, open awareness and participation in end of life discussions may be incongruent with the social, cultural and spiritual beliefs and practices of some ethnic minorities and faith groups. Moreover, people generally might not wish for information at all, in certain forms, or where it obfuscates emotion with fact, particularly in end of life care. For example, Innes and Payne (2009) suggest there may be a need to retain some degree of ambiguity as hope and realism may be incompatible with the provision of explicit information.

Disadvantaged information-seekers

How people access and use information varies and information-seekers are likely to be aged under 65, female, on higher income (Mayer et al., 2007). Nevertheless, some people—whether they are information-seekers or not—face particular challenges in obtaining information and therefore, access to service provision.

Worth et al. (2009) in a prospective longitudinal qualitative study notes the difficulties South Asian Sikh and Muslim patients face with regard to life-limiting illness and palliative care (e.g. institutional and personal racism, reduced awareness of hospice role and particular difficulties in discussing death). Other disenfranchised individuals such as people with learning disabilities–who are more likely to die before age 50 than someone who is non-learning disabled—consistently face unequal information and service access provision in the area of palliative care (O'Regan and Drummond, 2008). Nonetheless, tailored information on palliative and end of life care for disenfranchised groups is beginning to become more readily available through specific initiatives such as the Palliative Care for People with Learning Difficulties (www.pcpld.org) and specific projects such as 'books beyond words' (www.cancerhelp.org—using visual representations of palliative care). In turn, voluntary organizations such as www.cancerequality.org work towards addressing inequalities facing black and minority ethnic (BME) and refugee (BMER) communities by providing specific and sensitive information on cancer and palliative care while www.bmecancer.com—a social enterprise—raises awareness of cancer and related issues with the aim of empowering BME people to make informed choices.

Information-seekers and those who face barriers in seeking information constitute a range of individuals (patients, partners, family, friends, carers), profiles (gender, age, intellectual capacity), conditions (specific cancer, heart disease), disease stage (newly diagnosed, treatment, clinical trial, end of life), as well as specific needs (disabled, intellectual disability, ethnicity, sexual preference). Consequently, their needs, in *what form* the information is *presented or accessed* (written; leaflet/internet, audio-visual (DVD), verbal (internet, in person)), *who* presents it (doctor, nurse, other, carer, friend, family), and *when* (disease stage, setting; formal or informal) will vary considerably. Nonetheless, some aspects of information needs are relatively stable, e.g. patients generally value written information, personalized information is more likely to be shared with others and health care professionals are the most valued and utilized information resource.

Health care professionals, information, and communication

Currently, knowledge is accumulated much faster than it can be consumed and, somewhat ironically, this is true for health care professionals trying to keep up with the latest research, as much as patients who may attempt to glean condition-specific information from cyberspace. Information needs to be accessible, but it also needs to be comprehensible, timely, appropriate and useful. In any health care context, and specifically in the emotion-laden area of end of life care, a genuine therapeutic relationship is the fulcrum around which information should evolve and health care professionals are central to that.

Notably, the information age and the benefits it allegedly brings, has made previously sacrosanct information more widely available *and* accessible out with the formal environment of the clinical area. Moreover, patients' 'rights', patient autonomy, and patient-centred care is now embedded, in theory at least, in health care provision in the United Kingdom (UK). Consequently, the patient has *the right* to information previously the preserve of the 'monopolistic oligarchy' (Illich, 1997) of the medical fraternity. In the contemporary context, patients *expect* to be involved as an equal partner in decisions about their end of life care.

The move towards person-centred care and the emergence of the information age has therefore, intrinsically changed the patient-clinician relationship. Despite this and the increase in 'communication' research in health care interactions over the past decade, complaints about communication in the National Health Service (NHS) remain relatively stable.

Many complaints identify specific staff and highlight 'attitude and behaviour' and 'oral communication' as specific areas of concern. The prevalence and nature of these complaints suggests several things. First, communication is a key aspect of health care and when it is done badly it negatively impacts upon the patients' (and others') experience. Second, it may also suggest that patients, quite properly, have greater expectations of their health care experiences generally and with regards to their interactions with health care staff in particular. Third, patients clearly identify that 'communication' is an embodiment of numerous relational factors; interpersonal skills, personal attributes, e.g. attitude—as well as something more tangible such as information provision. Thus, it appears from the multiple areas of complaint grouped under the heading of communication, that patients perceive communication (noun) as something more than an act of simply conveying or transmitting information.

There are inevitably going to be challenges in working with patients who have access to potentially limitless information via the internet and in managing that within the evolving patient–clinician relationship in the complex and dynamic area of end of life care. To gain some understanding of these challenges it is worthwhile briefly reviewing how the patient–clinician relationship has evolved, particularly in relation to disenfranchised groups.

The patient–clinician relationship: a brief historical perspective

The patient–clinician relationship has changed significantly over the past six decades due to a number of factors: the changing role and roles of the health care professional, health care professionals' changing perspectives on the patient's role and their subsequent involvement in health care, and the increase in non-mainstream government health care initiatives or the self-help agenda. All of the above contributed to modernizing the patient–clinician relationship. Partnership is now generally preferable to paternalism and consequently, the context of communication and the how, where, who and why information and support is provided, has changed forever.

The previously omnipotent nineteenth-century medical physician has evolved markedly—none more so in the last 60–70 years and particularly over the past two decades. The emergence of the National Health Service and the hospice movement in the UK and their ongoing uneasy relationship with social and economic influences has significantly changed the role of the physician. In turn, new allied health professions have emerged alongside the developing nursing profession and so too have their roles and educational preparation. Health care is not the preserve of one profession but many—all with different roles and tasks that involve 'communication', information and support. Thus, the *changing role and roles of the health care professional* has evolved, and so too has their perceptions of the patient.

Patients have variously been presented as passive victims, survivors, active consumers, and latterly 'partners' (Pollock, 2005). The market economies introduced into the NHS under the Conservative government from 1979 to 1997 saw the notion of consumerism emerge, and thus previously passive patients became, in political rhetoric and sound bites, 'active consumers'. Medical advancement, changing health care delivery and funding, and the rise of 'celebrity' patients recounting their health care (often specifically cancer) experiences, as well as patients' groups (e.g. Gay Men Fighting AIDS) also influenced policy. *Perspectives on the patient's role and their subsequent involvement in health care* were irrevocably changed during that time and so too was their relationship with health care professionals.

For example, the emergence of Human Immunodeficiency Virus (HIV) in the mid-1980s saw clinicians having to engage with previously disenfranchised groups such as Injecting Drug Users (IDUs). These reluctant and peripatetic patients had to be engaged with, and maintained in, health care in order that HIV could be effectively combated, prevented, and treated. As a result, the locus of control within the patient-clinician relationship shifted to one that actively sought to accommodate the patient by recognizing their lifestyle choices or behaviours. This tacit recognition subsequently led the way to health and social care professionals being willing to work with disenfranchised groups and doing so in more innovative and pro-active *inclusive* ways.

An offshoot of the above was the emergence of what might be called *non-mainstream government health care initiatives* from the self-help/healing agenda that emerged in the early 1980s (including complementary and alternative medicines) to more recent initiatives such as 'positive psychology' and patient alliances. Patients therefore, increasingly wanted more than 'just' what was on offer from conventional medicine and were using computer-mediated communication to actively seek out that information and share it with others across the globe.

The former patient–clinician relationship was no longer appropriate, nor relevant, to modern health care. Subsequently, in some (Western) countries health care recognized that it needed to modernize its paternalistic approach to patients. This is perhaps best exemplified by the 'management' of infectious diseases, e.g. Directly Observed Therapy (DOT) for Tuberculosis in the 1960s. Patients were required by public health legislation to be confined to hospital and be observed taking their medication. More contemporaneous endeavours have attempted to 'encourage' recidivist HIV patients to take their anti-retroviral medications by emphasizing *partnership over paternalism*. Notably, terms evolved to more appropriately describe this shift and so patient *adherence* (to medication) became *concordance* (Wright, 2000).

Current policy directives now embrace the notion of a more equitable alignment of the patient–clinician relationship generally and specifically, with regard to communication.

The current policy and legal imperatives and associated initiatives

The relevant information and services policy context and initiatives in the UK advocate (a) better communication and information provision, (b) greater patient involvement in health care design, delivery, and research, (c) recognition of the importance of the patient experience plus its role in evaluating health care, (d) the patient's role as an expert or in relation to self-care and finally, (e) how information is used about patients.

Policy initiatives concerning the above are not necessarily end of life or cancer specific but address health care generally. Nonetheless, it is likely that the area of end of life care is where some of the greatest challenges with regards to communication, information and support will lie particularly with regard to ongoing discussions regarding euthanasia/assisted suicide/assisted dying. For example, from a broader population information perspective, the dying matters coalition (www.dyingmatters. org) set up by the UK National Council for Palliative Care in 2009, is committed to raising *public awareness* about death, dying, and bereavement and to stimulate debate. However, raising awareness of 'dying matters' unearths potentially controversial issues such as assisted dying—which may be viewed from a variety of perspectives in different countries. Dying and death affects everyone and anyone and individual per-spectives, economic, social, and environmental contexts, as well as religious leanings, vary considerably throughout the world. Nevertheless, even in our smaller localized and (arguably) developed spheres of practice and therefore, within a potentially less complicated context, there still remains considerable room for improvement with regards to communication *per se*.

In the United Kingdom the Cancer Reform Strategy (DoH, 2007), building upon the NHS Cancer Plan and its Scottish counterpart Better Cancer Care: An Action Plan (Scottish Government, 2008), both addressed key issues such as prevention, early diagnosis and better treatment. The Cancer Reform Strategy (DoH, 2007) highlighted the need for patients' information needs to be better addressed by the provision of quality information being made available to health care professionals *for use in face-to-face communication*. Thus, there was some recognition of the responsibilities of infor-mation provision *within* a patient–clinician relationship. Moreover, one of the goals of Cancer Research UK's 2020 campaign is that patients should receive bespoke informa-tion about their cancer at the point of diagnosis (Cancer Research UK, 2007).

Patients' research priorities

In turn, the Macmillan Listening Study (Corner et al., 2007) attempted to elicit patients' views about what topics should be researched as opposed to those currently being pursued by health care researchers. Notably, patients wanted to know how to live (and die) with cancer and with regards to communication, *how* best to communicate with partners and family about their diagnosis and treatment.

Spousal or partner involvement in health care interactions in cancer and palliative care is increasingly prevalent and recognized as an important aspect of treatment and care. Partner involvement adds to the complexity of these interactions and presents particular challenges for effective communication. The importance of health care professionals' actively facilitating patient-partner communication has been high-lighted (Hawes et al., 2006). However, no studies have investigated how and to what extent partner involvement in health care interactions in cancer and palliative care is currently facilitated. Thus, while policy directives and initiatives are laudable in expressing *what they want to happen* and are therefore, very prescriptive about what is expected—the Macmillan study demonstrates that the most important bit—the '*how to*'—*is often left unaddressed in practice*. Moreover, you could also argue that while the information needs (of patients) and information types or preferences (of patients) have been relatively well-researched, there has been considerably less, if any, attention given to *how* best to integrate information and support within the patient-clinician relationship–particularly within end of life care.

Data protection and freedom of information

There are two other key policy initiatives for health and social care professionals that it is important to briefly highlight from a UK perspective. First, is the Data Protection Act (DPA) (1998) and subsequent related legislation. This act requires that organizations manage information about individuals properly; e.g. securely, within time-limitations, non-transferably, accurately, relevantly, etc. It also gives individuals, e.g. patients, the right to know about information that is held about them and the accuracy or otherwise of that information. The Freedom of Information Act (FOI) (2002; www.ico.gov.uk; www.scotland.gov.uk) allows individuals to see information held about them and also other information about services that are provided by public authorities (e.g. care provision). The Freedom of Information Act works in tandem with the Data Protection Act and therefore some information may not be freely accessible. What both acts do is make organizations more publicly accountable for the information they hold, in ensuring its accuracy and, where appropriate, allowing it to be laid open to individual and public scrutiny.

The patient–clinician relationship: a moral imperative?

The patient–clinician relationship has therefore changed considerably over a relatively short period of time at the behest of various competing factors including policy directives, changing (professional and patient) roles, and associated perceptions plus heightened expectations of health care generally and communication in particular. The social, political, and economic context has been a significant driver in all of this, but so too has the desire of patients to bring about a more equitable and just patient–clinician health care relationship. It is therefore, important to note that it is primarily the patient and social and economic factors that have driven these changes rather than, arguably, any kind of moral imperative from Government or indeed, health and social care professionals.

This is important because, no matter how many politically correct policy directives governments or organizations issue regarding 'patient involvement', and no matter how many (skills-based) communication initiatives are implemented, it is professionals who have to be willing to engage with patients and embrace the notion of a therapeutic alliance. That is not to dismiss the influence of other contextual factors such as environment, workload, staffing, and resources, for example, all of which are very important and highly relevant in the current economic climate. Nevertheless, I would argue that health care professionals have to be convinced that genuine therapeutic engagement is *the right thing* to do and *the most effective way* of working with patients with regard to positive processes and outcomes. Otherwise, patients' desire for better 'communication' and information provision, and/or their disaffection with what is currently provided (e.g. quantity or quality of information and/or interaction), might lead them to seek out *alternative* sources of information and support.

The patient fights back: the rise of computer-mediated communications (CMC)

Albert Einstein (1879–1955) noted that *information is not knowledge*, while Sir Francis Bacon (1561–1626) asserted that *knowledge is power*. As such, it would be fascinating to know what both luminaries would have made of that modern phenomenon known as 'the internet'. The internet—computer-mediated communication (CMC)—has grown exponentially over the past decade. Unsurprisingly therefore, health and health care have not been untouched by this global phenomenon. Consequently there are an increasing number of studies on 'the internet' and its role in health care (e.g. Ziebland et al., 2004).

While 'the internet' may be a fertile ground for health care researchers, the more interactive, personal, and discursive aspects of CMC, such as blogs, are relatively unexplored. Yet, blogs may prove to be a fruitful area for exploring patients' unself-conscious and verbatim experiences. They may, arguably, provide a more naturalistic and contemporaneous view of the patient–clinician relationship, specifically around information needs.

Computer-mediated communications (CMC) and blogs

Millions of people throughout the developed Western world have access to computers and are increasingly computer-literate (AOL, 2005). Despite the popular image of the internet user as a geeky, young, web-obsessed male, older age groups are becoming increasingly conversant with a range of CMC from searching (Google), through trading (Ebay), social networking (Facebook), and latterly, blogging. Blogs emerged in the mid-1990s and there are an estimated 60 million blogs world-wide (Burrows, 2007). A blog, or a weblog, is an unsolicited online personal account that may be viewed and interacted with by others. It is frequently updated, author-driven, and reverse-chronologically ordered.

The prevalence of blogs exploded when free and easily accessible blogging engines such as LiveJournal and Bloggers emerged in 1999 (Blood, 2000). Currently, blogs are highly prevalent in politics via the phenomenon of participatory journalism—non-journalists who report and comment on current events. Corporate businesses have also been alerted to, and convinced by, the benefits of blogging—be it sharing stockmarket expertise or listening and responding to customers. Notably, while education has recognized the potential for blogs to enhance learning health care has, argu-ably, been less effective at realizing its potential contribution (Heilferty, 2009).

Blogs

The cornerstones of internet communication—speech, reach, anonymity, and inter-activity—are exemplified by blogs. The author may be relatively anonymous, and other 'advantages' include: the attenuation of physical distance, a concomitant reduced importance on physical appearance, plus a perceptible level of autonomy in terms of place and time.

An additional benefit of blogs generally not reported within the literature is the poten-tial for this medium to engage potentially socially isolated individuals with varying degrees of innate or acquired impairment. The increasing innovations within the Argumentative and Alternative Communication (AAC) field—high and low technolo-gies that compensate for (communicative) disabilities and thereby enhance communi-cative potential—may help previously disenfranchised populations to participate in interactive computer-mediated communities, such as blogs (Bryens, 2006).

However, there are potential drawbacks to blogging. Anonymity may be preferred but privacy may not be possible and non-restricted blogs can attract unwelcome 'posts'. Inaccurate information may be displayed on blogs and although blogs require minimal computer literacy they still require access to a computer. Moreover, some individuals may be more inclined to blog than others.

Who blogs and why?

Psychologists have reviewed the personality traits of bloggers primarily via young, 'healthy', undergraduate students (Guadagno, 2008). Consequently, the extent to which this literature is relevant to health care and end of life care is debatable. Nevertheless, one aspect of blogging that has consistently emerged as being unique and useful is the 'rant'—venting expression.

Illness narratives in life-threatening diseases have increasingly gained credibility as a means of accessing the patient's experience. Morgan et al. (2008) cite expressive writing as a way of coping in cancer care and this is corroborated elsewhere (Pennebaker, 1997). In turn, over 50 per cent of bloggers stated that they perceived blogging to be primarily a form of self-therapy (AOL, 2005). Understandably, there are therefore numerous cancer and life-limiting type blogs available—for a good example see www.ouramazingrose.blogspot.com, a blog written by the mother of a young girl with a rare life-limiting form of bone cancer. Blogs may therefore, offer a degree of agency where none exists to patients *and* carers, and as Gurak and Antonijevic (2008) suggest, as an expressive form, blogs may also assist in structuring experiences.

Blogs may be a more contemporaneous means of *author-driven* self-expression and information provision that is much more accessible, 'authentic', and interactive. Consequently, they may provide rich data on information needs and health care experiences.

CMC, blogs and their relevance for health care discourses

The diversity and potential empowerment of the internet has been lauded. Such 'diversity' has seen the emergence of informal, unofficial health-related internet sites and the accuracy of the information provided therein has been questioned (Huang and Penson, 2008). However, a study by Esquivel et al. (2006) found minimal inaccuracies, while Ilic et al. (2004) suggested that formal, professional sites were just as likely to house inaccurate information. Seale (2005) has also challenged the supposed 'diversity' of internet health care sites, noting that 'the [health care] internet' is now under the control of mainstream media (MSM). Consequently, Seale (2005) argues that gender stereotypes are still perpetuated (e.g. women need emotional support, men need information) and suggests any claim for unique expression is no longer valid.

Blogs are therefore relatively new phenomena that allow individuals to 'rant': make sense of their experiences and share those experiences with others. Blogs are important in that they provide an outlet and access to information sources *out with* the clinical encounter. Nonetheless, blogs are not an inclusive entity and certain groups are more likely to blog than others; and they are not without risk. Still, there is much that informal discourses such as CMC can tell us about communication, information, and support; what are we doing right and what we can do better? Accordingly, health and social care professionals should embrace these new technologies; use, adapt, and signpost them when and where appropriate. In saying that, CMC should only ever be an adjunct to, not a replacement for, authentic communication within the patient–clinician relationship.

From information, support and communication to human(e) interaction

As indicated previously, 'information', 'support', and 'communication' can be bland terms that might inadvertently lend themselves to being part of a box-ticking exercise. Similarly, as the quotation from George Bernard Shaw at the start of this chapter indicates, communication is often perceived as being an end-point rather than a process. Certainly, communication is often (magnanimously) recognized as being a 'two-way process', often involving a lot of listening, verbals and non-verbals—but other than that, it is still something we (allegedly) *do to others rather than take part in or perform as a nuanced interaction*. In some respects, you could argue that this perception of communication has some resonance with much that is wrong in modern nursing (and health care) today: the algorithmic approach to problem-solving and the concomitant lack of original and innovative thought; the tick-box culture supposedly evidencing 'professional accountability' but completely missing the point; the reduction of authentic human interaction to nothing more than a series of fragmented tasks undertaken by different people at different times, with different skills (and attitudes); a nominal engagement, and the perception that what is important is the skill and equipment—rather than the frightened, time-limited patient sitting in front of them.

In this chapter I have taken a constructivist approach to the topic of communication, information, and support. This view recognizes that individuals actively generate their own understanding and 'rules' are then used to make sense of their experiences, rather than accepting that communication, information, and support are passive things that health and social care workers do to, and for, others. Based upon the triumvirate of meaning, thought, and language—on meaning-making with a social context—this perspective recognizes the multiple realities of the people involved and the likelihood that these will change over time. At its core, therefore, is interaction between people and the *nuances* of these interactions; that these interactions are *actively performed* rather than passively dispensed (see McCreaddie, 2010; McCreaddie and Wiggins, 2009 on humour in health care interactions). Thus, teaching (cognitive-based) communication skills to health care professionals and providing good-quality written information are only small parts of a bigger picture. If you simply focus on individual aspects (skills, information needs) as a panacea for all problematic 'communication', then you risk reducing this complex and situated phenomenon to a series of mere tasks thereby stripping it of its innate humanity.

Of course, patients want quality information that is timely and appropriate and health care staff to be better skilled at meeting their needs. And why not? However, the rise in CMC and the haste with which patients have embraced this new phenomenon as well as the continuing prevalence of communication-related complaints suggests that we are still some way off getting this fundamental aspect of health care right—despite the evolving patient–clinician relationship and all the policy imperatives. Nevertheless patients still prefer to receive most of their information and support (and communication) from health care professionals: they want to be 'communicated with' but perhaps in a more symmetrical, individual, and engaging way. Moving towards a much broader conceptualization of communication as a *nuanced interaction* might encourage health care professionals to actively participate in such interactions and engage with patients, thereby bringing about a more authentic and therapeutic patient–clinician relationship.

Resources

♦ www.dyingmatters.org
♦ www.ouramazingrose.blogspot.com
♦ www.pcpld.org
♦ www.cancerhelp.org
♦ www.cancerequality.org
♦ www.ico.gov.uk
♦ www.scotland.gov.uk

References

Adams, E., Boulton, M., and Watson, E. (2009). The information needs of partners and family members of cancer patients: A systematic literature review. *Patient Education and Counseling*, **77**(2): 179–86.

AOL. (2005). America On Line survey says: People blog as therapy. http://media.aoltimewamer. com/media/newmedia/cb_press_view.cfm?release_num=55254441. Retrieved 20 Oct. 2010.

Blood, R. (2000). Weblogs: A history and perspective. *Rebecca's Pocket*. 7 Sept. 2000. Retrieved 20 Oct. 2010. www.rebeccablood.net/essays/weblog_history.html.

Bryen, D. N. (2006). Job-related social networks and communication technology. *Argumentative and Alternative Communication*, **22**(1): 1–9.

Burrows, T. (2007). *Blogs, Wikis, MySpace, and More*. Chicago: Chicago Review Press.

Cancer Research UK. (2007). http://aboutus.cancerresearchuk.org/who-we-are/our-goals/ goal-9-cancer-information/. Accessed 20 Oct. 2010.

Cappiello, M., Cunningham, R. S., Tish Knobf, M., and Erdos, D. (2007). Breast cancer survivors: Information and support after treatment. *Clinical Nursing Research*, **16**(4): 278–93.

Cassileth, B. R., Zupkis, R. V., Sutton-Smith, K., and March, V. (1980). Information and participation preferences among cancer patients. *Annals Internal Medicine*, **92**: 832–6.

Corner, J., Wright, D., Hopkinson, J., Gunaratnam, Y., McDonald, J. W., and Foster, C. (2007). The research priorities of patients attending UK cancer treatment centres; findings form a modified nominal group study. *British Journal of Cancer*, **96**(6): 875–81.

Data Protection Act 1998. (1998). London: Stationery Office.

Department of Health. (2007) *Cancer Reform Strategy*. London: Department of Health.

Duke, S. (2010). Communication skills training in end of life care 'Short of the mark?' *European Journal of Oncology Nursing*, **14**(4): 261–2.

Esquivel, A., Meric-Bernstam, F., and Bernstam, E. V. (2006). Accuracy and self correction of information received from an Internet breast cancer list: Content analysis. *British Medical Journal*, **332**(7547): 939–42.

Freedom of Information Act. (2002). London: Stationery Office.

Guadagno, R. E., Okdie, B. M., and Eno, C. A. (2008). Who blogs? Personality predictors of blogging. *Computers in Human Behavior*, **24**(5): 1993–2004.

Gurak, L. J. and Antonijevic, S. (2008). The psychology of blogging: You, me, and everyone in between. *American Behavioral Scientist*, **52**(1): 60–8.

Hawes, S. M., Malcarne, V. L., Ko, C. M., Sadler, G. R., Banthia, R., Sherman, S. A., Varni, J. W., and Schmidt, J., (2006). Identifying problems faced by spouses and partners of patients with prostate cancer. *Oncology Nursing Forum*, **33**(4): 807–14.

Huang, G. J. and Penson, D. F. (2008). Internet health resources and the cancer patient. *Cancer Investigation*, **26**: 202–7.

Heilferty, C. M. (2009). Toward a theory of online communication in illness: Concept analysis of illness blogs. *Journal of Advanced Nursing*, **65**(7): 1539–47.

Ilic, D., Risbridger, G., and Green, S. (2004). Searching the internet for information on prostate cancer screening: An assessment of quality. *Urology*, **64**(1): 112–16.

Illich, I. (1977). Disabling professions. In I. Illich, I. K. Zola, and J. McNight (eds), *Disabling Professions*. London: Marion Boyars Publishers, 11–39.

Innes, S. and Payne, S. (2009). Advanced cancer patients' prognostic information preferences: A review. *Palliative Medicine*, **23**(1): 29–39.

Mayer, D. K., Terrin, N. C., Kreps, G. L., Menon, U., McCance, K., Parsons, S. K., and Mooney, K. H. (2007). Cancer survivors information seeking behaviors: A comparison of survivors who do and do not seek information about cancer. *Patient Education and Counseling*, **65**(3): 342–50.

McCreaddie, M. (2010). Harsh humour: A therapeutic discourse. *Health and Social Care in the Community*, **18**(6): 633–42.

McCreaddie, M. and Wiggins, S. (2009). Reconciling the good patient persona with problematic and non-problematic humour: A grounded theory. *International Journal of Nursing Studies*, **46**(8): 1071–91.

Morgan, N. P., Graves, K. D., Poggi, E. A., and Cheson, B. D. (2008). Implementing an expressive writing study in a cancer clinic. *The Oncologist*, **13**(2): 196–204.

O'Regan, P. and Drummond, E., (2008). Cancer information needs of people with intellectual disability: A review of the literature. *European Journal of Oncology Nursing*, **12**(2): 142–7.

Pennebaker, J. W. (1997). Writing about emotional experiences as a therapeutic process. *Psychology Science*, **8**(3): 162–6.

Pollock, K. (2005). *Concordance in Medical Consultations: A Critical Review*. Oxford: Radcliffe Publishing.

Scottish Government. (2008). *Better Cancer Care: An Action Plan*. Edinburgh: Scottish Government.

Seale, C. (2005). New directions for critical internet health studies: Representing cancer experience on the web. *Sociology of Health & Illness*, **27**(4): 515–40.

Wright, M. (2000). The old problem of adherence: Research on treatment adherence and its relevance for HIV/AIDS. *AIDS Care*, **1**: 703–10.

Worth, A., Irshad, R., Bhopal, R., Brown, D., Lawton, J., Grant, E., Murray, S., Kendall, M., Adam, J., Gardee, R., and Sheikh, A. (2009). Vulnerability and access to care for South Asian Sikh and Muslim patients with life limiting illness in Scotland: Prospective longitudinal qualitative study. *British Medical Journal*, **338**: b183.

Ziebland, S., Chapple, A., Dumelow, C., Evans, J., Prinjha, S., and Rozmovits, L. (2004). How the Internet affects patients' experience of cancer: A qualitative study. *British Medical Journal*, **328**(7439): 564–67.

Chapter 6

Poverty and finance

Malcolm Payne

Poverty, social difference, health care, and end of life care

Poverty, the lack of financial resources to achieve an expected quality of life, is the most important factor in social difference. Differences in financial resources are associated with most differences among social groupings in any society: in education, health, housing, and community. Persistent patterns of financial difference create socio-economic groups in which power relations, social expectations, and culture connect with financial resources to lead to people forgoing social and health care because social exclusion makes it difficult for them to access services. Financial difficulties are important sources of stress. Dealing with the social impact of economic, and consequently social, differences between different groups in society is an important aspect of many kinds of social provision, including health care.

In particular, wealthier countries, wealthier regions, wealthier communities, and wealthier individuals are healthier and die later than their poorer equivalents. Since poverty is associated with ill health and early death, mortality, the rate of death in a population, is a marker of social difference. Any health care service therefore is concerned with responding to the impact of poverty in people's lives, because a disproportionate number of patients will be poorer rather than richer, and there will be connections between any ill health experienced by individuals and families and the many aspects of disadvantage associated with poverty. Because poverty is associated with early death, any service concerned with dying, death, and bereavement must respond to the loss of people's expectations: many patients and members of the public would have had a greater length and quality of life but for their poverty. As well as seeking to reduce the poverty that contributes to ill health, services need to respond to the social and personal consequences of poverty so that care can be accessed.

This chapter, therefore, argues that understanding and tackling poverty is an important aspect of end of life care, because it reduces social exclusion and forgone care. The report (CSDH, 2008) of a major commission of inquiry for the World Health Organization (WHO), chaired by Sir Michael Marmot, showed how health and ill health are, in important respects, socially determined. Its recommendations inform the WHO's overarching policy: to improve daily living conditions; to tackle the inequitable distribution of power, money, and resources; and to measure and understand the problem and assess the impact of action (World Health Assembly, 2009). These population-level interventions are distant from health care, yet they form the background of many actions to tackle health inequalities in countries across the globe, including the UK where Marmot has produced a similar document (Marmot Review, 2010). Health care services and policy on health inequalities have therefore shifted towards promoting more general social interventions on social determinants of ill health and unhealthy behaviours, to avoid adverse socio-economic factors accumulating over the life course to affect health (Davey Smith, 2003).

The WHO's policy on end of life and palliative care reflects similar social development objectives to its policy on the social determinants of ill health. The quality of life for the estimated 58 million people who die annually and their relatives can be improved by nations introducing palliative care services generally and pain control in cancer services (Stjernswärd, 2007).

The importance of poverty as a source of the inequality and social difference that underlies the social determinants of health inequalities suggests that health care services and policy need a stronger focus on understanding and responding to poverty; this is the focus of the next section. Because poverty is multi-dimensional, aligned with other forms of deprivation and inequality, it contributes to the social exclusion of particular groups from participation in society. This arises because people are unable to accumulate social and cultural as well as economic capital in their lives, within families and communities. As a result, interventions on health inequalities must tackle wide aspects of social exclusion, rather than focusing solely on health care services.

The final section examines the consequences of this analysis of social exclusion for end of life and palliative care. It reviews opportunities for interventions that can contribute to achieving international and national policies on poverty, social difference, and social exclusion and ensuring that services for dying and bereaved people are not forgone.

Poverty and deprivation: understanding and intervening

Poverty's connection with deprivation

How and why does poverty connect with so many social differences? The European Union definition of poverty helpfully covers most aspects that arise in debate:

> People are said to be living in poverty if their income and resources are so inadequate as to preclude them from having a standard of living considered acceptable in the society in which they live. Because of their poverty they may experience multiple disadvantage through unemployment, low income, poor housing, inadequate health care and barriers to lifelong learning, culture, sport and recreation. They are often excluded and marginalized from participating in activities (economic, social and cultural) that are the norm for other people and their access to fundamental rights may be restricted. (Council of the European Union, 2004: 8)

The first point is that poverty may refer to both income and wealth. Income is the periodic payments that people receive, usually as a wage from their employment or the payment of social security allowances. Wealth is the accumulated financial resources and property that people own. Income and wealth are to some extent substitutable. If people are wealthy, they can use their wealth in place of income; if they have a good income, they can save some of it to increase their wealth. Thus, discussions of poverty often refer to consumption, the capacity to consume goods and services, rather than income or resources; consumption counts both income and wealth.

The second point is that poverty may be absolute or relative. Absolute poverty refers to 'the lack of basic resources required for daily living—food, water, clothing, shelter . . .' (Shaw et al., 2007: 25). It is often defined in relation to an income threshold; the World Bank, for example, uses poverty lines of US$1.25 and $2.00 per day at 2005 prices for international comparisons. At this level, 1.4 billion people, 1 in 4 in developing countries, are in absolute poverty (World Bank, 2010). This number and the proportion have reduced markedly in the period from 2000 to 2005; however, the rising price of food has wiped out these gains. Relative poverty conceives of poverty as the EU definition does. It is defined by comparison with what is expected in a particular social environment. The social definition of relative poverty may refer to expectations in a particular country, or group of countries, a particular cultural milieu, or a particular age group.

The third point about poverty is that it leads to deprivation, that is, people in poverty are deprived of resources compared with other people. The deprivation may be material, for example people who have inadequate food, shelter or clothing, or social, for example lack of access to employment, health care, recreation, education, and social esteem.

Therefore, the fourth point about definitions of poverty such as the EU definition, is that poverty often leads to social exclusion, that is, a lack of access to social resources that come from participation in social and community life. In turn, the EU suggests, this may restrict their access to important human rights. Issues around social exclusion and inclusion are crucial to current understanding and debate about poverty.

Poverty in many dimensions

Multi-dimensional approaches bringing together lack of resources with the interaction of different dimensions of poverty and deprivation and their psychological and social consequences have become increasingly important (Jenkins and Micklewright, 2007: 8–11). Measures of socio-economic position are often combined in indices of multiple deprivation. All such measures show that poverty in any particular household is associated with many other deprivations. Deprivation is, in turn, associated with particular population groups: I review here minority ethnic groups and older people as examples.

Studies comparing different groups in several advanced societies show that ethnicity has an important impact on social difference (Medis Project, 2004). Platt's (2007) extensive literature review on poverty and ethnicity in the UK showed that all identified minority ethnic groups in the UK had higher rates of poverty than the population average. Bangladeshis, Pakistanis, and Black Africans suffered the highest rates, but Indian, Chinese, and other minority ethnic groups also had higher rates. Age groups that often experience poverty, for example children and older people, also experienced higher poverty than white people in the same age groups. The differences were apparent from various measures of deprivation, including income insecurity, lack of material goods, and duration of poverty. Bangladeshis were usually found to experience the greatest poverty. However, poverty was experienced differently by different groups.

For example, Bangladeshi and Indian people did not experience social isolation, while Black African and Caribbean people did. Ethnic differences arise across all forms of income, from employment, savings and assets and benefit income. Income from employment determines poverty, and this affects all ages, including retired people, whose income is affected by lifetime employment. Multi-generational households, common in Indian, Pakistani, and Bangladeshi communities, were affected by the resources of the whole family: older people's poverty comes from the whole house-hold's poverty. Therefore, end of life care services need to look at the position of the whole household, rather than just the individual patient or nuclear family.

More general information about older people comes from an extensive government review of research on older people's access to services, although research is limited (Just Ageing, 2009). Among general findings in relation to older people's health care are:

- ◆ Socio-economic inequalities favour people with higher incomes in all health care service areas, including primary care and especially specialist care and dental care.
- ◆ Socio-economic inequalities exist in the use of services with respect to income, ethnicity, employment status and education.
- ◆ Levels of utilization do not match levels of health need for the most disadvantaged groups.
- ◆ Poor people use GP services as much as and possibly even more than the better-off but this is not the case with specialists.

Studies of older people found that people from lower socio-economic groups were disadvantaged in specific services and studies of the total population found disadvantage in lower socio-economic groups that were particularly relevant to older people, including support to die at home. In social care services, wide discretion in services means that 'socio-economic inequalities are built in to the public social care system' (Just Ageing, 2009: 13). Older people also experience poor housing and neighbourhood facilities.

Forgone care arises where people do not make use of care that is potentially available (Allin and Masseria, 2009). The Just Ageing study identifies three major causes of inequality in health, housing, and social care as:

- ◆ Differences because some people did not recognize or accept that they needed services.
- ◆ Differences because some people were not aware that services were available.
- ◆ Differences in people's ability to make themselves heard and to navigate service systems (Just Ageing, 2009: 18).

These findings provide an agenda for practical action for service commissioners and providers, and is relevant to end of life care, since most people approaching the end of life are older people.

However, poverty and deprivation also affect health care service for younger people and families. Most state expenditure on benefits in kind in the UK (90 per cent) is provided through health and education services. Though poorer people benefit more from these and their benefit has increased in the past few years, 50 per cent of the increase in national income achieved in the ten years to 2009 went to the richest 20 per cent of the population and 40 per cent to the richest 10 per cent. So gains in a good economic climate went disproportionately to the rich (MacInnes et al., 2009). For example, Goldstein (2010) shows how excess mortality in childhood is closely related to the social context of poverty and inequality. The families of children who die young have different life experiences compared with better-resourced families. Family poverty increases when people have children, because parental employment or earning capacity often decreases, when people become unemployed and when people retire from employment. Therefore, policies that help families with the costs of maintaining children, that help people get into employment, or return to employment, and that help people remain in employment and generate earning capacity for as long as possible in the life cycle may be indicated (Jenkins and Micklewright, 2007: 11–12).

Studies also show that these multidimensional deprivations are an international phenomenon. For example, Kumar (1997), discussing Indian experience, suggested that inadequate facilities and poverty hinder treatment for cancer, which is generally detected late so most patients, incurable at diagnosis, are low priority for health care funding and there is no state-run social security system to support their families. A qualitative study of economic impacts of terminal illness in India (Emanuel et al., 2010) found that all patients and most informal caregivers had to give up work, all families had to sell property to support themselves and pay for medication and in most families children missed school. Rithara et al. (2009) describe the consequences of poverty for the families of women with breast cancer in an African village. Increasing poverty in the family forced them to sell property to fund treatment; this especially affects young mothers with dependent children. Most daily activities in the family cease, especially when patients become paraplegic, nearly half of patients become paralysed, increasing dependence on others, and half of patients' partners remarry and stop their financial support. By the time paralysis affects patients, family resources to pay for pain control medication have usually run out. De Simone's (2003) account of palliative care in Argentina identifies factors obstructing adequate end of life care. These include: increasing poverty, patients and families receiving inadequate information about their diagnosis or prognosis, drug availability and costs, and insufficient knowledge of the possibilities offered by palliative care by health care providers. Adejumbo (2009), referring to Nigeria, points to a high illiteracy rate, poverty, and poor health care infrastructure as making it difficult to implement palliative care services in ways that are similar to developed countries. Access to services, regular support and ability to use complex information are likely to be inhibited. Harding (2008) argues that although care for dying people may appear a low priority compared with other health care pressures, it is a moral entitlement to people in need of it.

All this evidence suggests that there is an important role for end of life care even in resource-poor nations. Also, end of life care services need to focus on the impact on the family's needs and resources, as well as health care objectives, if they are to help people to die well.

Deprivation, social exclusion, and social capital

The concepts of social exclusion and inclusion are connected with ideas about deprivation. Social exclusion draws attention to how disadvantageous social conditions cluster together and have social consequences, affecting the same groups in society.

In particular, poverty in income and wealth is often associated with physical divisions in cities, so that people experiencing poverty in consumption also experience poverty in their environment, and may cluster in particular areas (Byrne, 1999). If they suffer social exclusion in one aspect of life, they are likely to suffer it in other aspects. Poverty goes hand-in-hand with inequalities due to gender, race, disability and many other factors that lead to discrimination against particular groups in society.

However, social exclusion emphasizes social consequences rather than the factors in society that lead to the exclusion. So, instead of tackling poverty through better employment or social security, or ill health through better health services, we are led to worry about social integration. Emphasizing the idea of social exclusion may weaken personal and management responsibility to combat discrimination in organizational systems and workforces. It can also lead to 'blaming the victim', since there is sometimes a hidden assumption that people could do something about their own exclusion. Also, the idea of social exclusion may lead us to make assumptions that everything about people's lives will display problems. On the contrary, people who have poor general health because of poverty may have supportive family and community relationships, formed in the adversity that they have faced together.

Therefore, focusing on relative poverty, multidimensional deprivation and social exclusion raises questions about economic growth as a response to absolute poverty. Economic growth strengthens the capacity of economies to improve the lives and health of poorer people and is necessary but not sufficient for poverty reduction. Poorer nations and regions often have little choice in economic decision-making (Stiglitz, 2002: 268) and external interests of large multinational corporations determine events. Sen (1999) argues similarly that poverty comes from deprivation of the political and social freedoms to give people the capability to achieve a satisfactory life.

The economic evidence suggests, therefore that 'pro-poor' policies are needed to identify and change failures in the economy that exclude poor people from the opportunities that economic growth might bring them, to respond to social need and to benefit the well-being of poor populations. Accepting a political commitment to democratic freedom allows people to achieve beneficial social change and thus to avoid poverty and famine and is crucial to successful economic development. The World Social Forum (Fisher and Ponniah, 2003) suggested a range of areas of action to reduce inequalities within countries, and between countries and regions of the world. They emphasize democratic participation in decision-making about development as a right, since simple opposition to development may disadvantage poor people by preventing them from gaining its benefits. Cohesion and cooperation rather than competition, and openness and shared ownership rather than corporate structures are necessary. Page (2004), discussing the consequences of globalization for poverty, employment, health, and education, argues that as well as economic and political change, social policy should pursue the protection of citizens' and workers' rights, including rights to health and social care services such as end of life care. The Carnegie UK Trust Commission on the future of the UK civil society (2010) suggests four major areas of development for the future:

- There needs to be a more civil economy, so that economic development does not rely only on public or private sector investment.

- There needs to be a rapid and just shift to a low-carbon economy.
- Media ownership and content needs to be more democratic.
- Democracy needs to be more participative and deliberative.

Third sector developments, such as the hospice movement and palliative care, adapted to respond to local needs, can provide a useful counter-balance to adverse globalizing trends.

Responses to poverty and deprivation

The evidence and analysis about variation in the social and cultural capital available to households in poverty suggests helpful directions for social and health care policy and practice in responding to inequality and deprivation. Cultural capital is the capacity to understand and interpret the world around us in complex ways. People gain influence if they have secure and well-understood ideas about how to interpret the world, such as those offered by integration with community and minority organizations. Social capital is the power that we gain by having wide and supportive networks of relationships. Strategies for responding to the poorest people need to identify clearly the connections between poverty and its health consequences, identify barriers to health improvement, and set up strategies to deal with those barriers, as well as providing the necessary health interventions and developing better quality services. There needs to be a focus on the effective management and monitoring so that policies, planning and implementation of policy can achieve good-quality services provided in ways which overcome barriers to their use.

Strategies are also needed for participation, professional openness, and patient and family engagement in designing care for individuals and local groups that respond to trends towards impoverishment of particular localities or social groups. Inequality is not inevitable, but where it is a significant aspect of any society, it can be tackled by committed political action, which reduces social problems of all kinds in that society. Wilkinson and Pickett (2010) explored socio-economic inequalities in relation to a wide range of social and health care issues both between countries and within countries. They came to the conclusion that important health and social problems of the rich world are more common in more unequal societies. Wilkinson and Pickett (2010) conclude that everyone in a particular society benefits from equality. Exploring the pattern of rises and falls in inequality in particular societies, they also conclude that the political will to reduce inequality has consistently been shown to improve both equality and the significant social problems that arise from it.

Policies to tackle inequality directly, however, present many difficulties. There are two major approaches (Baker et al., 2009; Payne, 2010). Equal opportunities approaches accept that inequalities are inevitable, and seek to mitigate their effects, while diversities approaches seek to achieve equal outcomes by compensating for initial disadvantages and misfortune in people's lives and valuing diversities as positives for a society. Diversity approaches try to create conditions of life that are equivalent but appropriate to the differences in people. As with pro-poor policies on economic growth, an important way of doing this is for societies to recognize and support people's needs for participation and engagement with others. In particular, being an active part of society, being accepted by the people around us, being loved and supported and having the opportunity to love and support others recognizes important basic needs that all people experience. People also experience 'affective inequality' (Lynch et al., 2009) because the financial pressures in their lives reduce or remove the chances to have satisfying and secure relationships with others. Thus, justice is not just about the allocation of resources in society, or mutual respect, but the active incorporation of social and spiritual elements of life into more concrete services such as housing and health care. Such approaches have significant effects. For example, comparative study across several developed countries shows that more generous family benefits lead to lower child poverty, lower child mortality, and lower child injury mortality (Lundberg, 2009). In this way, general anti-poverty policies can have an impact on health inequalities.

End of life and palliative care interventions

This discussion suggests that poverty affects every society, but that every society benefits from greater equality and the reduction of health inequalities. Poverty reduction therefore needs to be part of the strategy of any social and health care service, including end of life and palliative care provision (Payne, 2010). This is for two reasons. First, in general, they are part of the social structure of societies that create poverty and inequality and need to play their part in combating those social impacts. Second, a service for dying and bereaved people must deal with the consequences of people's life experience of poverty and inequality in their society. Poverty and inequality also has a psychological, social and spiritual impact on people's lives that will have been interpreted differently through the cultural, religious, and spiritual imaginations dominant in different societies. This means that every service for dying and bereaved people will respond to poverty and inequality differently according to the cultural, social and spiritual experiences of the people they serve. End of life and palliative care offer an important opportunity for diversity and affective equality because it incorporates psychological, spiritual and social responses to need into delivery of social and health care services. Gallagher (2004) argues that 'financial pain' should be understood as an important aspect of 'social pain' affecting people who are dying and bereaved. He reviewed studies that show that financial worries affect the quality of life of people with chronic and terminal illness and contribute to psychological distress.

Consequently, end of life care services need to incorporate provision for responding to financial pressures in their work. Palliative care services can make two main responses: in their strategic management, with the long-term goal of reducing the impact of poverty; and in their services. Their strategy is the main way in which any organization takes steps towards the achievement of the ultimate goal of reducing the impact of poverty in society and on the lives of the people it serves. Such long-term goals need to be kept in corporate memory through developing policies and procedures that recognize it together with training and support to staff to enable them to develop their practice to include it. It must be part of the organizational culture and each individual's ethos in their work as an important objective. Formal statements of aims and policy, informal processes, and personal commitment must maintain its priority in the face of the immediate demands to dislodge it that always exist.

Since social inclusion is a significant factor in achieving diversity outcomes, an important strategy is to achieve participation by patients and their families in both clinical and service decision-making (Monroe and Oliviere, 2003). Both research and organizational opportunities to listen to patients and family members' voices can improve practitioners' understanding and help with the effects of poverty and inequality in the life experience that affects how they will respond to care and treatment. Support groups also generate considerable consumer satisfaction, with people feeling less alone, better understood, and more hopeful, and outcome studies demonstrate considerable quality of life benefits (Gottleib and Wachala, 2007). Emancipatory approaches to research and evaluation that use techniques such as group discussion and targeting specific groups potentially or actually excluded from participation in services are also important strategies. This contributes to evolving services so that they actively focus on poverty as an issue for services.

It is also important to identify aspects of service that create foregone end of life care. Ahmed et al.'s (2004) systematic literature review on access and referral to specialist palliative care identified three main practical barriers:

- ◆ Lack of knowledge, training and education among health professionals about palliative care and dealing with death and dying.
- ◆ Lack of standardized criteria to guide referral.
- ◆ People from socially excluded social groups and people with non-cancer diagnoses were not referred quickly enough.

Bestall et al.'s (2004) related qualitative research study looking at experiences of patients and professionals, suggested that many of these problems could be combated with more effective referral guidelines, better education, more widely-available effective home care services and effective support in care homes.

Service strategies in tackling exclusion are well-established in social work. Pierson (2002) identifies five main building blocks of a practice approach:

- ◆ Maximizing the income and working for the welfare rights (to receive full benefit entitlements and any discretionary benefits available) that individuals may have that are relevant in end of life care.
- ◆ Strengthening networks of relationships that will support individuals, for example by improving relationships and support received from families and communities, putting people in touch with people from whom they are estranged, encouraging and supporting potential informal helpers to begin, maintain, or enhance their care at the end of life.
- ◆ Building partnerships with services so that they are aware of and responsive to end of life issues. This is an important government strategy through the social care framework of the National End of life Care Programme (NEoLCP, 2010).
- ◆ Promoting participation recognizes that active involvement in decision-making about situations in which people need or provide care helps to achieve engagement and maintain commitment, and improve the quality of life of the people involved.
- ◆ Working in the neighbourhood, with organizations and individuals, to ensure that people are skilled in responding to end of life care issues, for example in

workplaces, schools and informal organizations that might support people facing end of life issues.

Palliative care services may need to strengthen their focus on end of life care for older people and on minority ethnic groups, since there is evidence that these groups experience general social exclusion, which may then affect the use that they can make of palliative care. Although death and bereavement may be expected among older people and the first consideration may be their health and social care, the financial pressures of illness, dying and financial reconstruction after the death of a family member on the surviving family may still be considerable.

The most well-established provision for dealing with poverty lies in the role of social work as part of end of life and palliative care in dealing with practical and financial problems (Reith and Payne, 2009). Financial issues are experienced at three stages of advanced illnesses: increased family costs during the period of treatment and care of the illness and palliative care, funeral costs and the costs of financial reconstruction during bereavement (Bechelet et al., 2008). Studies of palliative care patients show that they attach value to social workers who are able to deal with a wide range of practical issues and maintain consistent support over a period (Clausen et al., 2005; Beresford et al., 2007). As financial advice becomes more complex, end of life and palliative care services, rather than rely on non-specialized social workers, increasingly contract with specialist providers, such as Citizens Advice, law centres, or provide their own specialized welfare advice services. One audit of such as service (Levy and Payne, 2006) reports good outcomes, and an experiment in providing financial advice seminars for palliative care patients and families received good consumer feedback and was efficient in the use of staff time and other resources (Bechelet et al., 2008). An important element of this study was the range of issues that families of patients needed help with, including the extra costs of illness, social security benefits, retirement and pensions, funeral costs and costs of reconstructing family finances in bereavement. Help with pensions and financial services may need to call on a qualified independent financial adviser (IFA), registered with the Financial Services Authority. The arrangements for regulation of IFAs will change during the period 2012–15.

Conclusion

This chapter identifies poverty as a major source of social difference and of health inequalities and proposes that this is important for end of life and palliative care. Multi-dimensional consequences of poverty and deprivation are experienced differently in different population groups. Economic growth is not the whole answer to poverty, because development is uneven and poorer people cannot take advantage of economic opportunities. Therefore, pro-poor policies that advantage poorer populations and changes to economic systems that reduce inequalities and poverty and increase social inclusion are important strategies. Social and health care services such as end of life and palliative care have much to offer because they seek social inclusion alongside service provision. Services may be developed to achieve social inclusion and reduce forgone care and provide practical and welfare advice services.

Resources

◆ The Poverty.org website is an important source of statistical and policy information for the the UK, with links to international information: www.poverty.org.uk.
◆ The WHO website on the Social Determinants of Health, provides a range of
  resources, documents and an on-line course in implementing WHO policy on
  health inequalities: www.who.int/social_determinants/en/.
◆ The Inequalities blog provides useful information and regular updating on broader
  inequalities from both sides of the Atlantic: http://inequalitiesblog.wordpress.com.

References

Adejumo, A. O. (2009). Approaches in handling ethical challenges of cancer treatment and
  research in Nigeria. *African Journal of Medicine & Medical Sciences*, **38**(2): 15–20.

Ahmed, N., Bestall, J. C., Ahmedzai, S. A., Payne, S. A., Noble, B., and Clark, D. (2004).
  Systematic review of the problems and issues of accessing specialist palliative care by
  patients, carers and health and social care professionals. *Palliative Medicine*, **18**(6): 525–41.

Allin, S. and Masseria, C. (2009). Unmet need as an indicator of health care access. *Eurohealth*,
  15(3): 7–10.

Baker, J., Lynch, K., Cantillon, S., and Walsh, J. (2009) *Equality: From Theory to Action*.
  Basingstoke: Palgrave Macmillan.

Bechelet, L., Heal, R., Leam, C., and Payne, M. (2008). Empowering carers to reconstruct their
  finances. *Practice*, **20**(4): 223–34.

Beresford, P., Adshead, L., and Croft, S. (2007). *Social Work, Palliative Care and Service Users:
  Making Life Possible*. London: Jessica Kingsley.

Bestall, J. C., Ahmed, N., Admedzai, S. A., Payne, S. A., Noble, B., and Clark, D. (2004). Access
  and referral to specialist palliative care: Patients' and professionals' experiences. *International
  Journal of Palliative Nursing*, **10**(8): 381–9.

Byrne, D. (1999). *Social Exclusion*. Buckingham: Open University Press.

Clausen, H., Kendall, M., Murray, S., Worth, A., Boyd, K., and Benton, F. (2005). Would
  palliative care patients benefit from social workers' retaining the traditional 'casework' role
  rather than working as care managers? A prospective serial interview study. *British Journal
  of Social Work*, **35**: 277–85.

Commission of Inquiry into the Future of Civil Society in the UK and Ireland. (2010). *Making
  Good Society*. Dunfermline, UK: Carnegie UK Trust.

Council of the European Union. (2004). *Joint report by the Commission and the Council on
  Social Inclusion*. Brussels: Council of the European Union.

CSDH. (2008). *Closing the Gap in a Generation: Health Equity Through Action on the Social
  Determinants of Health. Final Report of the Commission on Social Determinants of Health*.
  Geneva: World Health Organization.

Davey Smith, G. (ed.) (2003). *Health Inequalities: Lifecourse Approaches*. Bristol: Policy Press.

De Simone, G. G. (2003). Palliative care in Argentina: Perspectives from a country in crisis.
  Journal of Pain and Palliative Care Pharmacotherapy, **17**(3–4): 23–43.

Emanuel, N., Simon, M. A., Burt, M., Joseph, A., Sreekumar, N., Kundu, T., et al. (2010).
  Economic impact of terminal illness and the willingness to change it. *Journal of Palliative
  Medicine*, **13**(8): 941–4.

Fisher, W. F. and Ponniah, T. (2003). *Another World is Possible: Popular Alternatives to Globalization at the World Social Forum*. Nova Scotia: Fernwood.

Gallagher, D. (2004). Finances. In D. Oliviere and B. Monroe (eds), *Death, Dying and Social Differences*, 1st edn. Oxford: Oxford University Press, 165–79.

Goldstein, R. (2010). Child death, poverty, and pediatric palliative care. *Journal of Pain and Symptom Management*, **39**(2): 351.

Gottleib, B. H. and Wachala, E. (2007). Cancer support groups: A critical review of empirical studies. *Psycho-oncology*, **16**(5): 379–400.

Harding, R. (2008). Palliative care in resource-poor settings: Fallacies and misapprehensions. *Journal of Pain and Symptom Management*, **36**(5): 515–17.

Jenkins, S. P. and Micklewright, J. (2007). New directions in the analysis of inequality and poverty. In S. P. Jenkins and J. Micklewright (eds), *Inequality and Poverty Re-examined*. Oxford: Oxford University Press, 3–33.

Just Ageing. (2009). *Socio-economic Inequalities in Older People's Access to and Use of Public Services*. London: Equalities and Human Rights Commission/AgeUK.

Kumar, S. (1997). The Calicut experience. *Hospice Bulletin*, **5**(3): 4.

Levy, J. and Payne, M. (2006). Welfare rights advocacy in a specialist health and social care setting: A service audit. *British Journal of Social Work*, **36**(2): 323–31.

Lundberg, O. (2009). How do welfare policies contribute to the reduction of health inequalities? *Eurohealth*, **15**(9): 24–7.

Lynch, K., Baker, J., and Lyons, M. (eds) (2009). *Affective Equality: Love, Care and Injustice*. Basingstoke: Palgrave Macmillan.

MacInnes, T., Kenway, P., and Parekh, A. (2009). *Monitoring Poverty and Social Exclusion 2009*. York: Joseph Rowntree Trust.

Marmot Review. (2010). *Fair Society, Healthier Lives*. London: author.

Medis Project. (2004). *Comparative Study on the Collection of Data to Measure the Extent and Impact of Discrimination within the United States, Canada, Australia, the United Kingdom and the Netherlands*. Luxembourg: Office for Official Publications of the European Communities.

Monroe, B. and Oliviere, D. (eds) (2003). *Patient Participation in Palliative Care: A Voice for the Voiceless*. Oxford: Oxford University Press.

NEoLCP. (2010). *Supporting People to Live and Die Well: A Framework for Social Care at the End of Life*. London: Department of Health.

Page, R. (2004). Globalisation and social welfare. In V. George and R. M. Page (eds), *Global Social Problems*. Cambridge: Polity, 29–43.

Payne, M. (2010). Inequalities, end-of-life care and social work. *Progress in Palliative Care*, **18**(4): 221–7

Pierson, J. (2002). *Tackling Social Exclusion*. London: Routledge.

Platt, L. (2007). *Poverty and Ethnicity in the UK*. Bristol: Policy Press.

Reith, M. and Payne M. (2009). *Social Work in End-of-life and Palliative Care*. Bristol: Policy Press.

Rithara, S. M, Kimani, G. G, Kirinya, D. (2009) The impact of breast cancer in a family and the community at large. *Supportive Care in Cancer*, **17**(7): 981–2.

Sen, A. (1999). *Development as Freedom*. Oxford: Oxford University Press.

Shaw, M., Galobardes, B., Lawlor, D. A., Lynch, J., Wheeler, B., and Davey Smith, G. (2007). *The Handbook of Inequality and Socioeconomic Position: Concepts and Measures*. Bristol: Policy Press.

Stiglitz, J. (2002). *Globalization and its Discontents*. New York: Norton.

Stjernswärd, J. (2007). Palliative care: The public health strategy. *Journal of Public Health Policy*, **28**(1): 42–55.

Wilkinson, R. and Pickett, K. (2010). *The Spirit Level: Why Equality is Better for Everyone*, rev edn. London: Penguin.

World Bank. (2010). *Overview: Understanding, Measuring and Overcoming Poverty*. Washington, DC: The World Bank. Retrieved 6 October 2010 from: http://web.worldbank.org/WBSITE/ EXTERNAL/TOPICS/EXTPOVERTY/EXTPA/0,contentMDK:20153855~menuPK:435040~ pagePK:148956~piPK:216618~theSitePK:430367,00.html.

World Health Assembly. (2009). *Reducing Health Inequities through Action on the Social Determinants of Health*. Sixty-second World Health Assembly, 22 May 2009, Agenda item 12.5 (Minute: WHA62.14). http://apps.who.int/gb/ebwha/pdf_files/A62/A62_R14-en.pdf (accessed 26 August 2009).

Chapter 7

Embracing diversity at the end of life

Heather Richardson and Jonathan Koffman

Introduction

Overall life expectancy is increasing in European and other developed countries, with more people living beyond 65 years of age. As part of population ageing, the pattern of diseases people suffer and die from is also changing. Given that many societies are now multicultural in nature, health and social care professions, regardless of setting, now require a different set of skills and knowledge to be able to ensure both equity and quality of health care provision for all. This situation is further amplified by growing numbers of older people from minority ethnic groups living in developed countries, which will continue to increase in coming years (WHO, 2004). The aim of this chapter is therefore to examine *differences that make a difference* among people when they negotiate institutions and practices for palliative and end of life care. This has particular resonance given that there is now increasing recognition of how multiple and simultaneous disadvantages can influence palliative care needs and end of life experiences (Koffman and Camps, 2008). In this chapter we provide the reader with an understanding of the current controversies with the language of understanding diversity in society. We then explore the experiences of advanced disease among Black and Asian Minority Ethnic (BAME) communities and related contributory factors. Finally, we offer a case study of a hospice based in an area characterized by social and cultural diversity, which has attempted to address issues of accessibility and acceptability of its services for the many communities it serves. The chapter draws on current evidence, primarily but not exclusively from the United Kingdom and the USA.

Race, ethnicity, and culture: semantic confusion

Race, ethnicity, and culture have potential to be presented as explosive concepts (Koffman, 2006). How these concepts are defined, and why ~~are~~ they are often conflated with other social metrics is often ignored within the medical literature. For the purposes of this chapter we understand race to be a classification of people on the basis of their physical appearance with skin colour the most popular characteristic (Fernando, 1991). In the past it has also been used as a way of dividing humankind which has denoted inferiority and superiority, linked to subordination and domination (Malik, 1996). Racialized research in science has a long and inglorious history (Gould, 1981). In the mid-nineteenth century, the cephalic index, a method for describing the shape of the skull, became a popular way of describing and dividing races. Under the influence of phrenology, a hierarchy of races was devised with white Europeans at the top and black Africans at the bottom. Intelligence, physique, culture, and morality were all placed in an order, the so-called 'Great Chain of Being' philosophy used to justify slavery, imperialism, anti-immigration policy, and the social status quo (Singh, 1997). Biological determinism also became prominent in medicine and medical practitioners frequently contributed to racialized science (Ahmad, 1993), with the theory of racial hygiene in Nazi Germany being a horrific and notorious example. However, differences that do exist between peoples and populations are very minor and largely reflect superficial physical characteristics such as facial features, hair, or skin colour. Researchers have therefore now discredited race as being an inaccurate and misleading concept.

Ethnicity, sometimes employed as a softer synonym for race, has been defined as: shared origins or social backgrounds; shared culture and traditions that are distinctive, maintained between generations, and lead to a sense of identity and group; and a common language or religious tradition (Senior and Bhopal, 1994). Ethnicity is fluid and depends greatly on context. For practical and theoretical reasons, the current preference is to permit the self-assessment of ethnicity (Senior and Bhopal, 1994).

Among other factors, culture underpins our ethnic identity. This too is a complex and problematic social phenomenon where a range of definitions exist. Culture is but one of several typologies of difference that has been used to signify diversity among individuals and groups. Narrowly defined from an anthropological perspective, culture can be thought of as that which refers to the '*patterns, explicit and implicit, of and for behavior acquired and transmitted by symbols, language, and rituals*' (Kroeber and Kluckholn, 1952). Seen as a 'recipe' for living in the world, this conceptual framework for culture explains the means of transmitting these 'recipes' to the next generation. However, this is a limited understanding of culture that, if used, risks minimizing discussions of cultural aspects of palliative care to an interpretive list of end of life beliefs and practices for a range of so-called 'cultural' groups. This has also been referred to as the 'fact-file' or 'checklist' (Gunaratnam, 2003) approach that, while informative in regards to interpreting behaviours, symbols, rituals, and other cultural practices of certain ethnic or religious groups that may be important and meaningful at the end of life, runs the risk of encouraging generalizations about individuals and groups based on cultural identity. This in turn may lead to the development of stereotypes, prejudices, and misunderstandings.

Differences that make a difference at the end of life

Demographic characteristics

Key demographic characteristics of the population that have been identified as influencing the need for palliative care include: age, gender, ethnicity/religion, socio-economic status, and household composition (Higginson and Koffman, 2005). Despite the broad relationships between demographic characteristics and the need for palliative care, there are inherent difficulties in the availability of comprehensive and usable demographic data on ethnicity to assess the palliative care needs of minority ethnic older people and to monitor services. This is because there are a range of factors, many of which are not fully understood, which affect service needs and how people use services. Emerging research suggests that there are two main factors which are of particular importance:

- ethnic differences in the patterning of diseases;
- culture and lifestyle differences and changes (which in turn have an effect upon disease and service needs).

It has been suggested that areas with high proportions of people from minority ethnic groups may need greater resources to train professionals to provide care to diverse communities as they will require 'an understanding of the different approaches taken by different cultures to end of life issues' (Tebbit, 2004: 12).

Professional and organizational influences

How we understand the influence of diversity in patterns of advanced disease, illness experiences, responses to treatment, and the use of specialist palliative care services is critical given increasing evidence that we are not all equal in death and dying (Crawley et al., 2000). Race or ethnic-based disparities in mortality and in diagnosis, quality of care, referral patterns to specialist palliative care, and treatments for pain and other physical symptoms have been documented in many developed countries (Crawley, 2005; Koffman et al., 2005). In the USA, a comprehensive review of evidence of unequal treatment commissioned by the USA congress and produced by its Institute of Medicine (IOM) documented race- or ethnic-based inequities in pain and chronic disease management, cancer care, and suggested that inequities may be due to patient-level, provider-level, and/or health system-level variables, alone or in combination (Smedley, Stith, and Nelson 2003). Patient-level factors would include ethno-cultural, social or other beliefs, preferences, or knowledge about health options. According to the IOM study, patient-level factors were thought to be the *least* likely contributor to disparities. On the other hand, both provider stereotyping and bias and how health care systems are organized, as well as the degree to which persons have access to care, were shown to more likely influence health outcomes for minority patients.

The existence of prejudice and stereotyping from the service provider's side of the exchange may be difficult for many non-minority providers to accept, as we all presume to consciously abhor such discriminatory attitudes and behaviours. The important contribution of the IOM report in thinking about this issue was its suggestion that it is not conscious attitudes that drive discrimination but rather those unconscious or implicit attitudes that may compel us when we are under duress.

Multiple disadvantage

Although there is a lack of data about people from minority ethnic communities, what is available demonstrates that some groups experience significant disadvantage during their lives (Ahmad and Bradby, 2007). Minority ethnic communities also experience a double disadvantage. They are more likely to live in materially and socially deprived areas and suffer all the problems that affect other people in these areas. Lastly, people from minority ethnic communities also suffer the consequences of overt and inadvertent

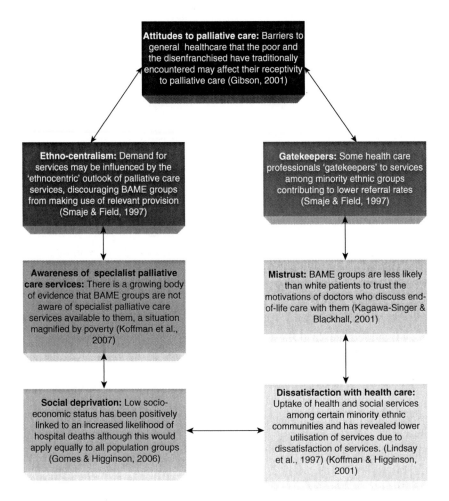

Attitudes to palliative care: Barriers to general healthcare that the poor and the disenfranchised have traditionally encountered may affect their receptivity to palliative care (Gibson, 2001)

Ethno-centralism: Demand for services may be influenced by the 'ethnocentric' outlook of palliative care services, discouraging BAME groups from making use of relevant provision (Smaje & Field, 1997)

Gatekeepers: Some health care professionals 'gatekeepers' to services among minority ethnic groups contributing to lower referral rates (Smaje & Field, 1997)

Awareness of specialist palliative care services: There is a growing body of evidence that BAME groups are not aware of specialist palliative care services available to them, a situation magnified by poverty (Koffman et al., 2007)

Mistrust: BAME groups are less likely than white patients to trust the motivations of doctors who discuss end-of-life care with them (Kagawa-Singer & Blackhall, 2001)

Social deprivation: Low socio-economic status has been positively linked to an increased likelihood of hospital deaths although this would apply equally to all population groups (Gomes & Higginson, 2006)

Dissatisfaction with health care: Uptake of health and social services among certain minority ethnic communities and has revealed lower utilisation of services due to dissatisfaction of services. (Lindsay et al., 1997) (Koffman & Higginson, 2001)

Fig. 7.1 Possible explanations to account for under-utilization of specialist palliative care among Black and Asian minority ethnic (BAME) groups.

racial discrimination—individual and institutional. The explanations to account for this, all of which may operate in combination, are highlighted in Figure 7.1 and have ramifications for wider public health policy. Identifying and eliminating health inequities in the delivery of quality palliative and related care therefore represents a critical mandate. Institutional standards for monitoring and ensuring the cultural sensitivity and competency of the palliative care workforce should be employed, as should strategies to increase community-based partnerships.

The special case of immigration: ramifications for palliative care services

Throughout human history, individuals, families, and groups have emigrated from their native homes to other places globally for many reasons: the prospect of education, economic, or social advantage; the need to escape war, oppression, torture, or other conflicts; or the desire to reunite with other family members. Globalization has brought with it an unprecedented increase in the numbers of persons who have migrated to developed countries. In 2005, there was an estimated 191 million immigrants world-wide: approximately 64 million of these immigrants arrived in Europe and 44 million in North America—a tripling of the immigrant populations in these regions compared to twenty years earlier. This trend is expected to continue and to increase. In the US, for example, it is estimated that by the year 2050, nearly two-thirds of the population will be immigrants.

The International Observatory on End of life Care, that monitors the global development of hospice and palliative care services around the world, reports that such services are unavailable or are uneven at best in under-developed and medium developed countries as compared to Europe and English-speaking countries (International Observatory on End of life Care, 2006). As a consequence immigrants may not have had much exposure to or knowledge of palliative care services provided by hospices or other health care institutions in their home countries. For example, the Observatory documented misperceptions about and stigmas regarding palliative care in Mexico. This findings has also been mirrored in the United Kingdom (Koffman et al., 2007). Expectations of palliative care may thus be lowered among minority ethic groups who bring from their country of origin misperceptions or lowered priorities for this type of care.

Arguably palliative care services which wish to increase uptake of their services by members of minority communities need to work to amend misconceptions and to raise expectations about how their services might support individuals at the end of life.

The experience of living with symptoms associated with advanced disease: the influence of ethnicity and culture

Symptoms, for example cancer-related pain, are never the sole creation of our anatomy and physiology. Rather, as Morris suggests, they emerge only at *'the intersection of bodies, minds and cultures'* (Morris, 1991). An appreciation of culture is important because it has potential to mediate the ways in which symptoms are identified and interpreted, how they are expressed, and how and in what ways people seek help.

Pain attributions and meanings are learnt by the members of a particular culture and then transmitted to others. This cycle of learning and expression is, by the very nature of culture itself, dynamic and fluid and was first observed in the classic study by Zborowski (1952) on pain responses of Italian-Americans, English-Americans and Irish-Americans, and Jewish people. English-Americans and Irish-Americans were stoical, whereas Jewish and Italian-Americans were more vocal about their pain, complaining about their discomfort. Zborowski predicted that ethnic differences would diminish through time as successive generations of immigrant descendents came to resemble the host culture.

Cancer-pain 'meanings' have frequently been identified as invoking religious beliefs. For example, recent research among black Caribbean and white British patients observed that attitudes to pain were mediated by religious beliefs that influenced attitudes towards medications and the accommodation of distress; cancer pain represented a test of religious faith and justified punishment (Koffman et al., 2008a). In this religious context, some black Caribbean patients believed that suffering was an expected part of life, to be endured in order to enter heaven (Koffman et al., 2008b). Although these findings may appear to be inappropriate and even anti-therapeutic from what is considered usual (Bendelow and Williams, 1995), health care professionals should remind themselves of Helman's three propositions about pain, all of which have resonance in the palliative care encounter:

◆ Not all social or cultural groups respond to pain in the same way;

◆ How people perceive and respond to pain, both in themselves and others, can be largely influenced by their cultural background;

◆ How, and whether, people communicate their pain to health professionals and to others, can be influenced by cultural factors. (Helman 2007: 185)

In other communities the actual language used to describe distress and suffering has implications for the delivery of palliative care. Krause revealed that the expression in Panjabi, 'Dil *me* girda hai', used by Panjabis in Bedford, often translates as the 'sinking heart' to reflect a range of psychological and somatic conditions (Krause, 2005). In addition, she suggests that the 'generalized hopelessness' which characterizes depressive disorders in women living in London would not be regarded as abnormal among Hindu, Muslim, and Buddhist women who would regard 'hopelessness' as an aspect of life which can only be overcome on the path to salvation. Ahmed (1998) takes the view that while South Asian patients may be well aware of their own psychosomatic symptoms, GPs (including Asian GPs) tend only to acknowledge physical symptoms but do not recognize psychological distress. The on-going challenge is for health care professionals to explore and acknowledge culturally determined understandings and expressions associated with advanced disease that do not mirror their own.

Religious and spiritual issues at the end of life

The experience of advanced disease can have a profound effect on patients and their family and friends. Indeed, during their illness many patients may raise questions that relate to their identity and self-worth as they seek to find the ultimate meaning in their life (Koffman et al., 2008b). Some patients attempt to answer these questions by examining their religious or spiritual beliefs. Formal religion is a means of expressing an underlying spirituality, but spiritual belief, concerned with the search for existential or the ultimate meaning in life, is a broader concept and may not always be expressed in a religious way. Speck suggests this usually includes reference to a power other than self, often described as 'God', or 'forces of nature' (Speck, 1998). This power is generally seen to help a person to transcend immediate experience and to re-establish hope. The importance of religion and spirituality among patients with advanced disease as a central component of physical and psychological well-being is increasingly recognized by health and social care professionals (Kearney and Mount, 2000). To this end, the acquisition of core competencies in the assessment and management of spiritual and religious care for specialist palliative care professionals has recently been highlighted within the National Institute for Clinical Excellence's (NICE) Guidance on Cancer Services (National Institute for Clinical Excellence, 2004).

Most of the published literature on the role of religious faith at the end of life are descriptive and focus on 'fact file' approaches to manage the experience of death and dying across different faiths (Neuberger, 2004). However, this approach is not without criticism as it has a tendency to over-categorize religious and cultural groups (Gunaratnam, 2003).

Grief and bereavement: socially patterned and channelled?

During this and the last century, we have greatly enlarged our understanding of the way people respond to the inner crises that are brought about by the death of a loved one. However, we have tended not to consider it adequately within its wider social and cultural contexts. Most of the early studies of grief and bereavement were conducted by psychiatrists on samples of white, invariably Christian widows (Parkes, 2001). This resulted in a very Western-centric view of what 'normal' grief comprised. Gorer's 1965 study of mourning customs in Britain suggested the social mores of southern England were deviant from other countries but he made no real attempt to establish the norm for the world. More recently, however, Rosenblatt and others have revealed that death is difficult for people everywhere. However, manifestations of grief in different cultures have been shown to vary considerably, since they were shaped by many cultural and religious factors (Rosenblatt, 1993). Each has its own approach for dealing with loss, which involved a core of understandings, beliefs, rituals, expectations, and etiquette. Approaches are developed to deal with the disposal of the body, the incorporation of death into religious ceremonies, the prescribed actions of mourning, and official remembrances.

Responding to difference: possible ways forward

The chapter, thus far, has described a variety of factors that influence the experience of people from BAME communities at the end of life and the care that they receive. The remainder of the chapter describes the approach of St Joseph's Hospice in East London which is working to improve accessibility and acceptability of its palliative care services for its population.

Introduction to St Joseph's Hospice

The population served by St Joseph's Hospice in East London is one characterized by diversity—including that which is ethnic in nature. Data from the 2001 census confirmed that BAME communities living in the local boroughs of Hackney, Newham, and Tower Hamlets accounted for 40.5%, 60.7%, and 48.5% respectively of their total populations. Projections of the same data for 2011 increase the proportion to 41.4%, 70.6%, and 49.4% respectively (Klodawski, 2009). The challenges of ensuring appropriate end of life care in this context are already documented. For example, Spruyt highlights problems experienced by patients with a life threatening illness and their carers from the Bangladeshi community living in East London arising from their ethnicity including communication difficulties, poor symptom control and serious financial problems (Spruyt, 1999). She also reports that at the time of her study there was no organizational commitment on the part of St Joseph's Hospice to ensure a model of care appropriate to the needs of this and similar communities. The work described in the remainder of this chapter is an attempt by the same organization to redress this gap.

In 2007 the hospice established a strategic plan which included an objective to engage proactively with its local communities. This work was deemed necessary following examination of data relating to service utilization in recent years, which suggested that uptake of hospice services was lower than might be expected by members of many of its local ethnic communities (Anderson, 2008). Those within the hospice were uncertain why. Speculation as to the cause identified possible concern around possible proselytization of non-Christians, anxiety as to whether cultural preferences would be met or even, more simply, lack of knowledge regarding the offerings of the hospice. Discussion as to how access to services might be improved for these marginalized groups was similarly ambiguous. The hospice realized that it needed to understand more about how members of the communities approached issues of death, dying and bereavement, their views of the hospice (if indeed they knew about it), and how they would like to see hospice services provided in the future if such care were to meet their needs and reflect their preferences. The Board of Trustees and the senior management team were in agreement that such work needed to be a priority if the hospice was to be accessible and acceptable to those who could benefit from its services locally. To this end financial resources and time were allocated to this piece of work which has spanned the subsequent four years to date. Such commitment by the Board and senior managers has proved invaluable and is evident in their on-going interest in the progress of this work.

At the outset the hospice recognized that long-term partnership with local ethnic communities was required to take forward suggestions for related service development and improvement. However, the means required to achieve this was less clear. Following some failed efforts on the part of the hospice to engage directly with these communities to discuss these questions further, the hospice sought the assistance of a local community development organization called Social Action for Health (SAfH) (see www.safh.org.uk for further details), with whom it has worked successfully to this end.

Working in partnership

The partnership with SAfH, has been key to establishing new links with previously excluded communities. SAfH is a well established local charitable organization working with marginalized communities towards health improvement and increased well-being. It encourages local ethnic communities to participate actively to achieve a state of well-being, to tackle related barriers and find solutions. Its underpinning principles include a commitment to work from the basis of peoples' own priorities and concerns and to encourage self determination around health and well-being. Previous work by SAfH had already confirmed concerns on the part of local people around the management of death in a culturally sensitive way.

The two organizations came together with the purpose of establishing a working interface between local ethnic community groups and the hospice. The principle aim of the work was to promote take up of the hospice services by members of local ethnic communities based on mutual learning and revised patterns of behaviour. The programme of work undertaken during the first three years of the partnership has been characterized by a number of shared operational aspirations including:

+ A commitment to prolonged engagement between hospice staff and local people as a basis for establishing meaningful and long-term relationships;

+ A commitment to engage in iterative discussion to understand the meaning and relative importance of comments made. It was hoped that such discussion would also facilitate a shared approach to the generation of ideas and solutions to address concerns or gaps in provision;

+ Use of stories as a basis for exploring peoples' views regarding care at the end of life and in bereavement and the relationship between these views and other aspects of their life including their history, culture and ethnicity;

+ A commitment to establish a reciprocal relationship between hospice staff and members from BAME communities. In practical terms this meant that the hospice would only expect to receive information and advice from local ethnic communities as long as it continued to respond in a considered manner to suggestions and requests for change;

+ Provocation of curiosity on the part of professionals to explore the differences between them and those they cared for. It was hoped that they would talk to each other about their heritage, their views of the world and their values.

The programme of work undertaken within the partnership has been an evolving one with changing aims and work plans. Such flexibility in approach can be viewed as a feature of community development and has enabled the programme to take new directions previously unanticipated. Whilst this flexibility has felt uncomfortable for the hospice at times because it has challenged the notion of establishing specific and fixed outputs and outcomes for the programme, it has proved essential to respond appropriately to differences between communities as well as within them. For example, work with the Turkish community in Hackney has had to follow a very different pathway to that pursued in engaging with the Bengali community in Tower Hamlets. The ability of SAfH to amend its methodology in response to the messages from its health guides is key to the success of the programme as a whole.

This work has been funded by the hospice, which, in turn, has sought grants from charitable sources to help meet related costs. On average, the hospice has paid in the region of £60,000 a year to SAfH for its contribution to the programme–a sizeable but worthwhile cost in the view of the hospice.

Community outreach

Community outreach has been the central and most constant feature of this engagement programme. SAfH uses an innovative approach to outreach by recruiting and training individuals from local ethnic communities to become 'health guides' (HGs). They work in their mother tongue with their communities to describe elements of health care provision, to encourage its uptake, explore resistance or anxieties and feedback to public service providers where appropriate. The HGs meet regularly as a group to share what they have learnt from their communities, to explore the meaning and implications for healthcare providers and to identify any gaps in knowledge. Their feedback, thoughts and ideas are subsequently discussed with the care providers, in the case of this project hospice staff, as a basis for service development.

In preparation for their work with the hospice, health guides were initially briefed on the range of work and philosophy of hospice. The HG's remit was a specific focus on end of life care and bereavement support issues within different community groups. Discussions between health guides and the different community groups were rarely limited to a single issue, often extending over a number of meetings, the subject matter revisited and refined each time. Showing a willingness to revisit and refine discussions on the part of the HGs helped to build trust and confidence about hospice care among the different ethnic groups.

The learning on the part of the health guides was fed back into the hospice through formal and informal meetings. In addition meetings of members of the local ethnic communities and hospice senior staff were arranged through SAfH at which key concerns were raised, often reinforcing issues previously raised by health guides. The meetings were always well attended by local people as they were seen as an opportunity to tell their story and influence plans for service improvement. Those participating were vocal and confident in their views, assisted by health guides and other facilitators working with them in their own language. These meetings and other open exchanges proved useful on two accounts—for the hospice in its efforts to tailor services to the needs of the different communities and also for local people who were reassured that that they were being listened to and their views respected. Very often significant relationships were forged between professionals and members of the public who took part—which have served as important platforms for on-going dialogue subsequently. Where difficulties were encountered in making the change these would be explained to local community groups and an alternative solution proposed.

Dialogues

Initial discussion between health guides and members of local ethnic communities identified some recurrent areas of concern related to their religious beliefs, spiritual needs, and cultural rituals, which the hospice needed to explore further. Such understanding would form the basis for delivering services that were responsive to such preferences, and thereby acceptable to the different groups.

By way of example, engagement with local Somali and Bengali people had identified three key areas about which they had sufficient concern to make them reticent about using the hospice. They were:

◆ How news that death is imminent is conveyed without causing offence;
◆ The nature of home care services, and how professionals can help families avoid crises associated with the end of life care at home;
◆ The role and treatment of relatives at the end of life.

A series of conversations or dialogues were established to discuss openly and resolve concerns and this process proved successful and acceptable for both parties. The process may be viewed as confirmation of the value of dialogue as a means of breaking down barriers, helping those involved to understand the rationale and position of others in relation to issues of concern. It also demonstrated the commitment of the hospice to deliver culturally sensitive care, which was probably the evidence that encouraged the different community groups to use the hospice in future with more confidence.

Staff education and training

Staff at the Hospice were, in the main, keen and committed to provide culturally sensitive care to all the different community groups. However, gaps in their understanding and knowledge were evident. For example, at the start of the programme staff would often question the need for change particularly in relation to access, given that hospice services were often running at full capacity, albeit underused by people from local ethnic groups. Staff also described a lack of confidence about how to address issues of ethnic difference and described concerns about doing the 'wrong thing' to people with whom they did not share a common language, history, or cultural norms.

Education and training for staff was therefore deemed essential right from the start in order to increase awareness around the best ways to achieve culturally sensitive care among different ethnic groups served by the hospice.

The aim of the training was to build the confidence of hospice staff members to address such differences—to ask people what they wanted, to clarify any areas of ambiguity, and to encourage discussion with family members and other caregivers about how the care by the hospice could be amended further to meet individual cultural or ethnic preferences. The training also sought to challenge previously held perceptions regarding the needs of specific community groups, achieved by providing new information regarding their views about end of life care, gained through related conversations. These often confirmed a multiplicity of views with intergenerational differences, as well as serving to clarify the cultural and ethnic derivations of the some of the most strongly held preferences. As a result, the hospice has seen a new confidence in many of its staff in relation to working with new communities, accompanied by an increasingly flexible approach to patient care. The training was provided at both formal and informal levels, through multi-disciplinary discussion as well as to different professional groups and across the different teams within the hospice, including those that are non-clinical in nature.

Engagement and training of volunteers

Volunteers have become increasingly important contributors to the process of engagement between the hospice and its local communities. Like many hospices, volunteers at St Joseph's Hospice are well established members of the workforce providing assistance with a whole range of functions spanning care, hospitality, administrative support, creative arts, and similar.

It became evident fairly early on in the programme that existing volunteers could be co-opted onto the programme to help the hospice establish stronger relationships with its local ethnic communities. Volunteers, who came from particular communities were encouraged to partake in new training that would give them skills to listen to stories on the part of their peers, and to talk to them about the work of the hospice and their involvement in it. Training was also provided in the use of creative arts as a basis for establishing discussion around issues of death and bereavement and helping people explore their emotions. The creative approach known as 'The Colours of Life' [see Resources] has been widely used by volunteers and staff alike with support and supervision.

Over the last three years new volunteers have also been proactively recruited specifically to work on the programme of engagement. SAfH has, at times, led such recruitment—focusing on particular communities traditionally under represented within the hospice. In addition, a significant number of people have since become volunteers, having been introduced to the hospice by health guides or through other elements of the outreach programme. Consequently, the number and make up of the volunteers has changed significantly over the last three years, and is increasingly representative of the local communities served by the hospice. These volunteers are arguably one of the most vital resources available to the hospice as it continues to work towards a service which is accessible and acceptable to the different local communities. They often serve as ambassadors raising the hospice profile. They welcome new patients in their own language and with an awareness of their preferences arising from a shared culture. In addition, through their own knowledge and established role within the hospice, they help guide professionals within the hospice to redress aspects of their care or the environment of the hospice that have been off-putting or unacceptable to people from particular local ethnic or cultural groups in the past. In so doing, they assist in the process of achieving cultural competence. During 2010, the number of volunteers working at the hospice has increased by nearly 50 per cent, including 28 new volunteers recruited and trained to run the Colours of Life workshop. The ethnic profile of the volunteers has also changed—only half now identifying themselves as UK White. The volunteers delivering the Colours of Life workshop are, in the main, from BAME communities, working with local groups that include African Caribbean, Turkish, Kurdish, and Bengali people. Informal feedback regarding the experience and development of both volunteers and participants has been encouraging and the majority of the new volunteers have been retained.

Social engagement

A smaller but significant element of the programme has been the infrequent opportunities for meetings between hospice staff and local ethnic communities. These events which take place at least annually are carefully facilitated by SafH—providing an opportunity for participants to talk to each other about their history, life experiences and plans for the future. SAfH and the local people provide the hospitality—extending an invitation to hospice staff to join them. These events include refreshment, conversations, information, and entertainment that reflects the culture of the groups hosting the event. They are illuminating in this respect, often beautiful and create new interest in the culture of the group on the part of the hospice staff who attend.

The events are essentially informal in nature and are well attended by local people as well as hospice staff. They have proved highly valuable in providing a pleasurable reason for many local ethnic communities to visit the hospice who would otherwise be very uncertain or 'frightened' to do so. Their role as hosts is also an empowering one, creating a different dynamic between them and the staff in the hospice who would normally be their carers. From attending, many people express a wish to return to the hospice as their expectations had been positively changed by the experience. Staff, similarly, report increased comfort about working with these communities and a new confidence about engaging with them at an individual level. Review of data relating to care provided at St Joseph's Hospice confirms that as a result of these various activities people from different ethnic groups are increasingly comfortable to use the hospice and indeed do so. By way of example, in 2006–7, only 19% of in-patients were from BAME communities. In the first 8 months of 2010, this number has increased to 33%; BAME patients under the care of the community palliative care team is higher still at 43% of the total.

Reflections on the programme as a whole

To date this programme of engagement has been restricted to a relatively small number of communities, and will need to be replicated many times to reach out to the different and changing communities in the area. Whilst the scale of the task presents something of a challenge, it is a process that becomes easier each time—as the hospice draws on its growing and transferable skills of listening to stories communicated via health guides or similar who can work in their mother tongue.

Conclusion

The palliative care movement has assumed a leading role in addressing the health and social care needs of patients and families facing the inevitability of death. It has only been recently that attention has focused on the importance of providing care for the increasingly diverse societies in the developed countries. This has now become a demographic imperative. This chapter has shown that the language of understanding difference is complex yet fascinating. When considering its influence in the provision of care at the end of life and during bereavement, we must hold two lenses simultaneously. Understanding and serving the needs of specific communities requires us to apply a framework of equity of provision. Yet at the same time, however, we must not lose sight of the individuals and families before us, whose needs and concerns may not conform to preconceived or stereotyped patterns. At the end of life, an individualized approach to care with a focus on quality is paramount for any patient, regardless of their ethnic or cultural background.

Resources

- Publications on the website of Social Action for Health (www.safh.org.uk) regarding its work in East London related to community development. Specific publications of possible interest include:
  - The report on Managing Death in the Muslim Community in Tower Hamlets. Improving After Life Services (2007).
  - Engaging in Dialogue (2009).
  - The Colours of Life handbook (2010).
  - Anderson, W. (2008). *Responding to need: St Joseph's Hospice and the population it serves*. London: St Joseph's Hospice.

References

Ahmad, W. I. U. (1993). *'Race' and Health in Contemporary Britain*. London: Open University Press.

Ahmad, W. and Bradby, H. (2007). Locating ethnicity and health: Exploring concepts contexts. *Sociology of Health and Illness*, **29**(6): 795–810.

Ahmed, T. (1998). The Asian experience. In R. Salman and V. Bahal (eds), *Assessing Health Needs in People from Minority Ethnic Groups*. London: Royal College of Physicians.

Bendelow, G. A. and Williams, S. J. (1995). Sociological approaches to pain. *Progress in Palliative Care*, **3**: 169–74.

Crawley, L., Payne, R., Bolden, J., Payne, T., Washington, P., and Williams, S. (2000). Palliative and end-of-life care in the African American community. *Journal of the American Medical Association*, **284**: 2518–21.

Crawley, L. M. (2005). Racial, cultural, and ethnic factors influencing end-of-life care. *Journal of Palliative Medicine*, **8**(1): ss58–69.

Fernando, S. (1991). *Mental Health, Race and Culture*. London: Macmillan.

Gibson, R. (2001). Palliative care for the poor and disenfranchised: A view from the Robert Wood Johnson Foundation. *Journal of the Royal Society of Medicine*, **94**: 486–9.

Gomes, B. and Higginson, I. J. (2006). Factors influencing death at home in terminally ill patients with cancer: Systematic review [see comment]. *BMJ*, **332**(7540): 515–21. [Erratum appears in BMJ **332**(7548): 1012.]

Gorer, G. (1965). *Death, Grief and Mourning in Contemporary Britain*. London: Cresset.

Gould, S. J. (1981). *The Mismeasure of Man*. Harmondsworth: Penguin.

Gunaratnam, Y. (2003). Culture is not enough., In D. Field, J. Hockey, and N. Small (eds), *Death, Gender and Ethnicity*, 1st edn. London: Routledge, 166–86.

Helman, C. G. (2007). *Culture, Health and Illness*, 5th edn. London: Hodder Arnold.

Higginson, I. J. and Koffman, J. (2005). Public health and palliative care. *Clinics in Geriatric Medicine*, **21**: 41–5.

International Observatory on End-of-life Care. (2006). *Global Development*. Lancaster: IOEC, Lancaster University.

Kagawa-Singer, M. and Blackhall, L. J. (2001). Negotiating cross-cultural issues at the end of life: 'You got to go where he lives'. *JAMA*, **286**(23): 2993–3001.

Kearney, M. and Mount, B. (2000). Spiritual care of the dying patient., In H. Chochinov and W. Breitbart (eds), *Handbook of Psychiatry in Palliative Care*. New York: Oxford University Press, 357–93.

Klodawski, E. (2009). *GLA 2008 Round Ethnic Group Population Projections*. Data Management and Analysis Group, Greater London Authority, London.

Koffman, J., Morgan, M., Edmonds, P., Speck, P., and Higginson, I. J. (2008a). Cultural meanings of pain: A qualitative study of Black Caribbean and White British patients with advanced cancer. *Palliative Medicine*, **22**: 350–9.

Koffman, J. (2006). The language of diversity: Controversies relevant to palliative care research. *European Journal of Palliative Care*, **11**(1): 18–21.

Koffman, J., Burke, G., Dias, A., Ravel, B., Byrne, J., Gonzales, J., and Daniels, C. (2007). Demographic factors and awareness of palliative care and related services. *Palliative Medicine*, **21**(2): 145–53.

Koffman, J. and Camps, J. (2008). No way in: Including the excluded at the end of life. In S. Payne et al. (eds), *Palliative Care Nursing: Principles and Evidence for Practice*, 2nd edn. Maidenhead, UK: Open University Press, 362–82.

Koffman, J., Donaldson, N., Hotopf, M., and Higginson, I. J. (2005). Does ethnicity matter? Bereavement outcomes in two ethnic groups living in the United Kingdom. *Palliative and Supportive Care*, **3**: 183–90.

Koffman, J. and Higginson, I. J. (2001) Accounts of carers' satisfaction with health care at the end of life: A comparison of first generation black Caribbeans and white patients with advanced disease. *Palliative Medicine*, **15**(4): 337–45.

Koffman, J., Morgan, M., Edmonds, P., Speck, P., and Higginson, I. J. (2008b). 'I know he controls cancer': The meanings of religion among Black Caribbean and White British patients with advanced cancer. *Social Science and Medicine*, **67**: 780–9.

Krause, I. (2005). The sinking heart, a Panjabi communication of distress. *Social Science and Medicine*, **29**(4): 563–75.

Kroeber, A. L. and Kluckholn, C. (1952). *A Critical Review of Concepts and Definitions*. Vol. *47*. Cambridge, MA: Peabody Museum of Archaeology and Ethnology, Harvard University.

Lindsay, J., Jagger, C., Hibbert, M., Peet, S., and Moledina, F. (1997). Knowledge, uptake and the availability of health and social services among Asian Gujarati and white persons. *Ethnicity and Health*, **2**: 59–69.

Malik, K. (1996). *The Meaning of Race: Race, History and Culture in Western Society*. Basingstoke: Palgrave.

Morris, D. (1991). *The Culture of Pain*. Berkeley: University of California Press.

National Institute for Clinical Excellence. (2004). *Guidance on Cancer Services: Improving Supprtive and Palliative Care for Adults with Cancer*. London: National Institute for Clinical Guidance.

Neuberger, J. (2004). *Dying Well: A Guide to Enabling a Good Death*, 2nd edn. London: Radcliffe Publishing.

Parkes, C. M. (2001). A historical overview of the scientific study of bereavement., In M. S. Stroebe et al. (eds), *Handbook of Bereavement Research: Consequences, Coping and Care*. Washington, DC: American Psychological Association, 25–47.

Rosenblatt, P. C. (1993). Cross-cultural variation in the experience, expression and understanding of grief. In D. P. Irish, K. P. Lundy, and V. J. Nelson (eds), *Ethnic Variation in Dying Death and Grief: Diversity in Universality*. Washington, DC: Taylor and Francis, 19.

Senior, A. and Bhopal, R. (1994). Ethnicity as a variable in epidemiological research. *British Medical Journal*, **309**: 327–30.

Singh, S. P. (1997). Ethnicity in psychiatric epidemiology: Need for precision. *British Journal of Psychiatry*, **171**: 305–8.

Smaje, C. and Field, D. (1997). Absent minorities? Ethnicity and the use of palliative care services, In J. Hockey and N. Small (eds), *Death, Gender and Ethnicity*. London: Routledge, 142–65.

Smedley, B. D., Stith, A. Y., and Nelson, A. R. (2003). *Unequal Treatment: Confronting Racial and Ethnic Disparities in Healthcare*. Washington, DC: National Academies Press.

Speck, P. (1998). Spiritual issues in palliative care. In D. Doyle, G. W. C. Hanks, and N. MacDonald (eds), *Oxford Textbook of Palliative Car*. Oxford: Oxford University Press, 805–814.

Spruyt, O. (1999). Community-based palliative care for Bangladeshi patients in east London: Accounts of bereaved carers. *Palliative Medicine*, **13**: 119–29.

Tebbit, P. (2004). *Population-Based Needs Assessment for Palliative Care—A Manual for Cancer Networks*. London: National Council for Hospice and Specialist Palliative Care Services.

WHO. (2004). *Better Palliative Care for Older People: The Solid Facts*. Milan: World Health Organization Regional Office for Europe.

Chapter 8

Disability and the death and dying agenda

Carol Thomas

Introduction

This chapter considers the interests of disabled people in the social management of death and dying. There is much to cover: the meaning and nature of disability, including key concepts; the social position and health status of disabled people across the globe; the relevance of disability for end of life care (EOLC) services and practice; and principles for the avoidance of inequity in the provision of support at the end of life.

Disability: a review

What is disability?

Disability is a global human phenomenon that has been much studied in recent decades (for example, Bickenback et al., 1999; WHO, 2010). As the World Health Organization (WHO) explains, disability concerns the interaction between bodies and their environments. Individuals whose bodies are impaired[1] from birth, or acquire impairments during the life-course, interact with social arrangements and physical landscapes that disadvantage them in comparison to their non-disabled brothers and sisters. Whatever their global setting, disabled people face social barriers that threaten life and/or undermine their ability to flourish. Disabled people must survive impairment effects and develop the capacity to overcome disablism (in some societies the concept *ablism* is used interchangeably with *disablism*). Because understanding these concepts is a way into thinking about end of life care, the following definitions are set out in some detail, and used throughout this chapter (elaborated in Thomas, 1999, 2007):

> *Disablism*: the *social* imposition of *avoidable restrictions* on the life activities, aspirations and psycho-emotional well-being of people categorized as 'impaired' by those deemed 'normal'. Disablism is social-relational in character and constitutes a form of social oppression in contemporary society—alongside sexism, racism, ageism, and homophobia. As well as enacted in person-to-person interactions, disablism may manifest itself in institution-alized and other socio-structural forms. Disabled people have struggled against disablism both individually and collectively—the latter under banner headlines such as 'the social

---

[1] Impairments are those bodily differences or variations that carry medical meanings denoting 'pathology', 'disease' or 'abnormality'.

model of disability' (Oliver, 1996) and 'nothing about us without us' (Charlton, 1998). The 'medical model' of disability is opposed because it assumes that the problems and troubles faced by disabled people are entirely caused by their impairments. In individual lives, disablism always interacts with other dimensions of social disadvantage or advantage associated with social identity—for example, gender and 'race'.

Impairment effects: the *direct* and *unavoidable* impacts that impairments (physical,[2] sensory, mental health, intellectual) have on individuals' embodied functioning in the social world. Impairments and impairment effects are always bio-social in character, and may occur at any stage in the life-course.

Disability across the globe

In this section, we explore the intersection of patterns of morbidity and mortality among disabled people with their social conditions—in different parts of the globe. This helps to place their 'needs' for end of life care, alongside the need for other forms of health and social support, in context.

In the resource-rich regions of the world, most societies have reached a stage of development wherein: (i) a large and growing proportion of disabled children and adults now survive into old age, and (ii) the ageing of the non-disabled population means that a large and growing proportion of society's disability is found among old people—as the chronic diseases of old age take their toll (especially cancers, cardiovascular and neurological conditions). In Britain in 2010, for example, the Office of Disability Issues estimated that 50 per cent of the 10 million disabled people are over state pension age (65 years; ODI, 2010); a large proportion of old people eventually or invariably present to medicine with co-morbidity and complex needs (Marmot, 2010). At the other end of the age scale, technological developments mean that the survival of babies and infants with 'severe' and often 'life-limiting' impairments (physical, sensory, and intellectual) is an increasing reality for parents, care services, and, later, the education system (DoH, 2008; Priestley, 2003).

Disabled people of all ages are among the most economically disadvantaged and socially excluded layers in society (Oliver and Barnes, 1998; Priestley, 2003; Thomas, 2007). Living in conditions of relative poverty is the lot of most families with disabled children and disabled adults—especially the old (Roulstone and Barnes, 2005). In some regions, notably Eastern Europe, the institutionalization of disabled people is still a reality—especially children and adults with intellectual impairments. However, a feature of democratic resource-rich societies today is that several decades of struggle by the organizations of disabled people and their allies have advanced claims to equal rights and social justice. Campaigning for independent living—that is, freedom from institutional and professional control—has been a priority for disabled people's movements in richer nations (ibid). Independent living arrangements can enable disabled people to take control of their own lives by having the ability to make meaningful choices about the nature and quality of their support services. Bringing this into reality requires legislative mechanisms whereby money is paid directly to disabled people

---

[2] Physical impairments include chronic and infectious diseases—as well as congenital impairments and accidental injury or trauma.

(e.g. 'direct payments', 'personal budgets') rather than channelled through social or health services. Active support and community living for people with intellectual disabilities is the preference where support needs are much greater (People First, 2010).

In North America, Europe, and Australasia there are now important government legislative and policy commitments to the full equality and social inclusion of disabled people. For example, in the United States (US) the Americans with Disabilities Act (ADA) was passed in 1990, designed to challenge discrimination and bestow equal rights to a disadvantaged minority. In Britain, the Disability Discrimination Acts (1995, 2005), the setting up of the Disability Rights Commission (DRC Act, 1999), and the introduction of legislation facilitating Direct Payments (1996) and Individual Budgets (Welfare Reform Bill, 2009)—all appeared to be ushering in a new century of disability equality, inclusion and self-governance. In 2004, the British Prime Minister's Strategy Unit promised that disabled people should have full opportunities and choices to improve the quality of life and to be treated as respected and equal members of society (Cabinet Office, 2004: 7). Moreover, the *Equality Act* (2010) is now in force in Britain, bringing disability anti-discrimination law into alignment with equality legislation covering other groups in need of protection—on the grounds of race, gender, age, sexual orientation, or religious belief. However, the degree to which there is a match between the fine words emblazoned in legislative/policy commitments and the reality of life on the ground for disabled people is another matter altogether, as we shall see below.

Turning to the global South, to the resource-poor regions of the world, living with impairment effects and disablism is of a different order: basic subsistence and perilous survival are the realities for millions of disabled children and adults, especially in war-torn countries and depleted rural locations (Priestley, 2001; Barnes and Sheldon, 2010). The World Health Organization informs us that 80 per cent per cent of the world's growing disabled population (estimated at 650,000) live in low-income countries and have limited or no access to basic services, including health and rehabilitation facilities (WHO, www.searo.who.int/en/Section1174/Section1461.htm, accessed Nov. 2010). The impairments involved are typically: infectious and chronic diseases (especially HIV and AIDS), injuries, violence, malnutrition, and other causes closely related to poverty. Accidental injuries are regular occurrences (typically traffic accidents, drowning, falls, burns, or poisoning) and acts of disablist violence are endemic in many resource-poor communities (especially child and female-partner abuse, youth violence, war and conflict) (ibid.).

In this context, impairment effects and disablism interact seamlessly in the lives of individual disabled children and adults, and the struggle of the majority in conditions of absolute poverty is relentless and often hopeless. The priority is for access to basic health and rehabilitation services, followed by access to education and employment, but these services and life-course opportunities are often minimal or almost entirely absent, especially in rural areas (Tomlinson et al., 2009). Where health care and rehabilitation services are available in middle-income countries with developed urban centres, disabled people find that their access to services is disadvantaged by physical and attitudinal barriers among service providers, together with a shortage of mobility devices and other assistive technologies (Tomlinson et al., 2009; Officer, 2010).

If access is possible, then the tendency to medicalize individuals' disability makes its appearance—echoing traditions in Western medicine. Additional social barriers operate forcefully in more favourable economic circumstances in relation to education, employment, transport systems, housing and the built environment (Barnes and Sheldon, 2010).

None the less, wherever possible disabled people have actively resisted their degradation in the resource-poor world. Indeed, the disabled people's movement has formed, wherever conditions permit, and is now international in scope—see, for example, the websites of the Disabled People's International and the International Disability Alliance. In part, this internationalism follows from globalization—the increasing interconnectedness of individuals, groups and communities within worldwide economic, political, and cultural networks. The pressure for equality exerted by the disabled people's movements across the globe has certainly been felt by governments and international agencies. In 2007, most governments signed up to the United Nations Convention on the Rights of Persons with Disabilities (2006)—a very important international agreement about protecting and promoting the rights of disabled people throughout the world. The Convention requires governments to take action to remove barriers and give disabled people real freedom, dignity and equality. The fifty-eighth World Health Assembly called upon WHO and its Member States to work towards ensuring equal opportunities and promoting the rights and dignity of disabled people, especially those who are poor. Countries are requested to strengthen national policies and programmes on disability, including community-based rehabilitation services. However, it must not be forgotten that some 20 million people with disabilities currently lack mobility devices to participate and become independent in society. Access to mobility devices is a vital human rights issue, as highlighted by Article 20 of the UN Convention (Officer, 2010). It is also of note that the WHO is soon to release a landmark World Report on disability and rehabilitation across the globe.

Health inequalities

The sketch above indicates that encounters with death and dying among disabled people are commonplace in childhood and young adulthood in resource-poor regions. In the economically advanced nations, disabled people increasingly face death and dying in older adulthood or at the start of life when survival is compromised by serious foetal or birth-related impairment. Despite this stark global variation, it remains the case that mortality rates among disabled people exceed those of the non-disabled in all societies—and at each stage in the life-course (WHO, 2008). This takes us into the realm of research on the social determinants of health and health inequality (Marmot, 2010). Recent research in this area among disability studies scholars and social epidemiologists has demonstrated conclusively that disabled children and adults are at *excess risk* of developing poor health—because they are at excess risk of living in poor socio-economic circumstances (Emerson et al., 2009; Marmot, 2010). This is summarized in an important list of findings derived from an extensive literature review submitted to the *Strategic Review of Health Inequalities in England Post 2010* (the Marmot Review) (Emerson et al., 2009).

Findings: disability and health inequality

◆ Disabled people experience significantly poorer health outcomes than their non-disabled peers, including in all aspects of health that are unrelated to the *specific* health conditions associated with their disability. Poorer health outcomes are also experienced by the carers of disabled children and adults.

◆ There are strong social gradients, across the life-course, in the prevalence of disability.

◆ These gradients are likely to result from a combination of factors including:

  • *The impact of adversity and disadvantage on the onset of health conditions associated with disability.*

  • *Intergenerational transmission of socially patterned health conditions associated with disability.*

  • *The impact of disability on social mobility.*

◆ As a result, disabled children and adults are more likely than their peers to be exposed to general socio-economic conditions that are detrimental to health. A significant proportion of the risk of poor health of the disabled person themselves and carers appears to be attributable to their increased risk of exposure to socio-economic disadvantage.

◆ Some health conditions associated with disability or impairments may specifically impede the attainment of positive health.

◆ In addition, disabled children and adults are at risk of experiencing social exclusion and discrimination associated with their disability (disablism). The direct effects of such discrimination on health include reduced access to appropriate health care. Indirect effects of such discrimination on health operate through increased social exclusion, restricted social mobility, and the psychological impact of direct personal experience of disablist actions. (Reproduced from *Strategic Review of Health Inequalities in England Post 2010* (Emerson et al., 2009).)

Expressed succinctly: (a) disabled people live with excess *primary risks* of worsening morbidity and premature mortality associated with their impairment/impairment effects, and (b) if life progresses, disabled people are exposed to excess *secondary risks* of morbidity and mortality associated with the impact of disablism on lived experience— especially poverty (absolute or relative). It is crucial that health professionals understand these dynamics if they are to deliver accessible and effective health care: preventative, curative, and end of life. Of particular note are the 'complex conditions' and 'complex needs' presented by children and adults exposed to secondary risks.

End of life care (EOLC)–meeting needs

Care at the end of life

It is no surprise that services offering end of life care are unavailable luxuries to the vast majority of disabled people in resource-poor regions (IOELC, 2010). The urgent priority identified by the World Health Organization (WHO) is the improved availability and accessibility of primary and secondary care services, and access to rehabilitative services (Tomlinson et al., 2009). The WHO guidelines on Community Based Rehabilitation (CBR) are viewed as key tools for 'disability and development' (Officer, 2010). CBR began as a network of grassroots practitioners who work with disabled people and their families to promote functioning and participation, but since 2004 the focus has shifted from an exclusive concern for medical rehabilitation and assistive technologies (prostheses, wheelchairs, etc.) to a wider strategy designed to promote equalization of opportunities, poverty reduction, and social inclusion (WHO et al., 2004). The updated guidelines advocate the inclusion of people with disabilities in areas such as education, livelihood, and political participation. It is of note that some 20 million people with disabilities currently lack the mobility device they need to participate and become independent in society; thus access to mobility devices is a vital human rights issue, as highlighted by Article 20 of the UN Convention on the Rights of People with Disabilities (Officer, 2010). Of particular relevance here is the insistence that WHO guidelines and policies are now developed in partnership with the disabled people's movement—in line with the social model of disability and the slogan 'nothing about us without us' (Oliver, 1996; Charlton, 1998).

Turning to Europe, North America, and Australasia we find a different scenario. End of life care services, and international EOLC agencies, have certainly developed apace since the 1980s (see other chapters in this volume). However, these services remain largely inaccessible to disabled children and adults—whose needs are often complex for the reasons outlined above (Priestley, 2003; Stein, 2008; Stein and Kerwin, 2010). Expressed another way, it can be argued that EOLC services have developed historically with 'normal adults' in view, especially 'normal adults with cancer' (Clark and Seymour, 1999; Payne et al., 2008). In Britain today, for example, cancer services remain a top priority for the National Health Service (NHS) because cancer continues to account for one quarter of all deaths (DH, 2007; NICE, 2004: 3). It is only in the recent Cancer Reform Strategy (DH, 2007) that social inequalities in cancer have been addressed head-on: readers will find that a whole chapter is devoted to 'Reducing Cancer Inequalities'—with explicit reference to inequalities associated with disability, as well as socio-economic status, gender, sexuality, and ethnicity. It is also acknowledged in the Strategy that there is a need for *equality sensitive research* to advance understanding of patients' and carers' experiences of living and dying with cancer—to inform health service planning and delivery (DH, 2007: 24). Indeed, it must be remembered that active carers are often disabled people too.

Of course, unintended disablism can take many guises in health and EOLC service planning and delivery in resource-rich nations (Priestley, 2003; Fisher and Goodley, 2007; Stein, 2008; Stein and Kerwin, 2010). As noted in the definition above, disablism is often enacted in person-to-person interactions as well as manifesting in institutionalized and other socio-structural forms. For example, the well-meaning 'help' offered by health professionals may actually prove to be 'unhelpful' to disabled people (Thomas and Curtis, 1997). Thus, obvious areas for scrutiny are: i) the bricks and mortar of services—i.e. the accessibility and suitability of hospitals, hospices, care homes, and private residences, etc., ii) the availability of necessary medical practices and specialist equipment, and iii) the policies and individual attitudes and practices of providers (Koffman and Camps, 2004). Detailed studies are required to uncover the ways in which disablism may manifest itself in specific EOLC settings and contexts, but a good example is Runswick-Cole's research in Britain on the care of disabled children (Runswick-Cole, 2010, see also Ryan and Runswick-Cole, 2008). As part of a wider study, she reports on qualitative interviews with three mothers of disabled children with life-limiting or life-threatening impairments. It was found, in short, that the families experienced systematic attitudinal and economic disadvantage:

> [The mothers and children] face isolation in the home, from families and friends, while at the same time receiving unsatisfactory support from service providers . . . Disabled children with the most complex forms of impairments and their families experience the most complex forms of disablism as they face marginalization in the wider community, from friends and family and even from other parents of disabled children who succumb to the 'direarchy' of impairments. (Runswick-Cole, 2010: 824)

The legacy of profound disablism: Not Dead Yet

No chapter on disability and death can ignore the fundamental fears left in the minds of disabled people by the genocidal practices visited upon their kind in the twentieth century, most notably in Nazi occupied territories during the Second World War (Friedlander, 1995; Priestley, 2003). Research is increasingly uncovering the gruesome reality: that the medical profession in Germany supported and assisted in the extermination of thousands of disabled people in the concentration camps—people with a wide mix of impairments (physical, sensory, mental health, intellectual). The medical rationale was that a disabled life was a life of lesser value, indeed, a life *not worth living*. This *lesser value* philosophy has cast long shadows forward. It was originally elaborated in the eugenics movement—a movement that spread across Europe and North America in the early twentieth century (Priestley, 2003). Eugenicists set up programmes for the mass sterilization of disabled people so that the 'degeneration' of the population could be prevented (Shakespeare, 1998).

Space prevents the further exploration of this theme but it must be mentioned here because it explains the hostility and fear displayed by many disabled people and their allies toward medicine and 'end of life care'. There has been particular hostility, in recent years, to debates in Britain about making medically *assisted suicide* legal; and disabled people in parts of the world where assisted suicide is practised are often fearful of *any* forms of end of life care. Not surprisingly, the spectre of *lives not worth living* haunts these debates, and disabled people's movements have campaigned against assisted suicide using the slogan Not Dead Yet. Given this history and context, the time has not yet come, for many, to consider lobbying for the *right* to a good death for disabled people.

It is important to understand that these themes relate to another disablist practice that was widespread in the twentieth century in the West, and now has a bearing on disabled people's exclusion and anxieties about end of life care. This is the 'warehousing' of disabled people in large-scale residential institutions—a medically authorized (sometimes driven) practice, often labelled as 'care', begun in the nineteenth century (Borsay, 2005). Indeed, one of the most important subjects in the study of disablism is understanding the control that health and social care professionals exercised, past and present, in the daily lives and destinies of adults and children with impairments and 'mental illness'. It can be argued that principal among professionals who continue to exercise control are doctors—located at the apex of a professional hierarchy that includes nurs-es, occupational therapists, physiotherapists, social workers, and teachers and psy-chologists in the 'special needs' sector of education. This history has had at least two important effects on a societal scale—both of which impact upon EOLC. First, during the nineteenth and twentieth centuries, social structures and behaviours in towns and rural communities developed with only the 'normal', 'able-bodied', person in view. This shaped and consolidated a material environment and set of mainstream social institutional arrangements and practices fit only for the non-disabled (Thomas, 2007). Second, health and welfare professionals became key social forces in promulgating and sustaining (often unconsciously) the ideological mantra that people with impairments are *dependent* individuals, that is, people 'in need' who can only 'take from' rather than 'give to' society, and whose individual disadvantage is believed to be directly attributa-ble to the 'pitiable' condition of 'being impaired'. Such ideas quickly became culturally normative (Oliver, 1996). It is not surprising, therefore, that disabled people have waged a long and difficult struggle for independent living and self-autonomy. This his-tory must be taken into account when opening up EOLC services to disabled people.

Principles for the avoidance of inequity in the provision of end of life support services

Service Planning and Practice

Given the information about disablism and impairment/impairment effects intro-duced in this chapter, it follows that those involved in end of life care service planning and delivery are encouraged to turn their minds to the principles and duties set out in relevant national and international anti-discrimination and equality legislation, not least the United Nations Convention on the Rights of Persons with Disabilities (2006). It is useful to reproduce Article 25 of the Convention—and to ask readers to consider its implications for the provision of end of life support services specifically, in their own spatial and social contexts:[3]

Article 25
Health
States Parties recognize that persons with disabilities have the right to the enjoyment of the highest attainable standard of health without discrimination on the basis of disability. States Parties shall take all appropriate measures to ensure access for persons with disabil-ities to health services that are gender-sensitive, including health-related rehabilitation. In particular, States Parties shall:
(a) Provide persons with disabilities with the same range, quality, and standard of free or affordable health care and programmes as provided to other persons, including in the area of sexual and reproductive health and population-based public health programmes;
(b) Provide those health services needed by persons with disabilities specifically because of their disabilities, including early identification and intervention as appropriate, and

[3] Observant readers will have noticed that I am now using the phrase *end of life support services*—dropping the word 'care'. This phrasing sits more comfortably with all that has been said.

services designed to minimize and prevent further disabilities, including among children and older persons;

(c) Provide these health services as close as possible to people's own communities, including in rural areas;

(d) Require health professionals to provide care of the same quality to persons with disabilities as to others, including on the basis of free and informed consent by, inter alia, raising awareness of the human rights, dignity, autonomy, and needs of persons with disabilities through training and the promulgation of ethical standards for public and private health care;

(e) Prohibit discrimination against persons with disabilities in the provision of health insurance, and life insurance where such insurance is permitted by national law, which shall be provided in a fair and reasonable manner;

(f) Prevent discriminatory denial of health care or health services or food and fluids on the basis of disability. (Reproduced from United Nations Convention on the Rights of Persons with Disabilities (2006), www.un.org/disabilities/default.asp?navid=13&pid=150; accessed Nov. 2010.)

It also follows that another requirement of service planning and provision is that, wherever possible, disabled people must have a voice in procedures, and the opportunity to participate meaningfully—and in keeping with the variety of needs and perspectives involved. That is, the principle *nothing about us without us* should apply as much to end of life service provision as it does to services that operate to support disabled people at other moments in the life-course. However, *extra* sensitivity is required because disabled people—both collectively and individually—may be reluctant to engage in matters of death and dying for the historical reasons sketched out above.

If sensitivity and respect *for difference* are clearly in evidence in social interactions at the end of life, most disabled adults can feel more confidence in revealing that they have long been the *experts* when it comes to the everyday management of their own bodies and conditions—or at least have some expert knowledge. This lays the foundations for collaboration between service providers and users in end of life support.

Looked at from another angle, service planners and providers may benefit from approved Disability Equality Training (that is, quality training run by disabled people) or the study of disablism and impairment effects in national and international contexts (Stein, 2008; Stein and Kerwin, 2010). The latter would also include the development of knowledge about the social epidemiology of the health states and health inequalities involved (see the Marmot Review 2010 in the UK).

Some suggested resources:

◆ Read international publications and Web resources in Disability Studies—for example: the free Archive texts held by the Centre for Disability Studies, Leeds University, UK: www.leeds.ac.uk/disability-studies/archiveuk/index.html. (All sites accessed Nov. 2010.)

◆ Seek out special resources—for example: The Independent Living Institute: www.independentliving.org/indexen.html; the Deaf Wellness Centre at the University of Rochester Medical Centre, US: www.urmc.rochester.edu/deaf-wellness-center/; the Canadian Centre on Disability Studies: http://disabilitystudies.ca/; *Source*: the international information resource centre on health and disability:; and People

First: www.peoplefirstltd.com/. The Center for Practical Bioethics has useful 'case study' resources of relevance: www.practicalbioethics.org/.

Case study

We end with a case study that combines experiences outlined in a disabled woman's life narrative, gathered in my research with disabled women, with *fictional* end of life experiences drawn from insights in my research on cancer patients' death and dying in the UK (Thomas et al., 2004). This individual case is designed to pose some questions for readers, bearing in mind all that has been written above, especially:

- what needs does Helen's position present to end of life support services?
- how can these best be met?
- and what other considerations come into play?

Helen, aged 66

Helen's cerebral palsy means that she is a wheelchair user with no verbal speech. She describes herself as severely disabled. To communicate, she has a word board on a tray. She has recently been diagnosed with terminal cancer.

As a child and younger adult (until her mid-30s): Helen lived mainly at home with her caring parents—who encouraged as much 'normally' as possible. She did spend a few years in residential 'special' schools or Care Homes—but she hated the way that these were run on institutional lines. She recalls in her writing: '*I observed everything was done to a strict routine, and at the convenience of the staff. Residents were helped to get up in the morning at a certain time. Meals were eaten in a large communal dining room, residents requiring assistance in going to the toilet could only go at certain times in the day—and woe be tide you if you were caught short, and all residents had to be in bed by a specific time . . . I came back to my family home depressed. I thought I had glimpsed the inevitable life I would lead in a Home when my parents could no longer look after me . . . I used to beg my parents to allow me to enter a Home just to get the dreaded business over with. However, my parents didn't listen to my pleas, and I am mighty glad, as the future has turned out very different from the one I imagined*'.

Independent living in middle-age: Helen's parents helped her to establish her future living arrangements whilst they were in sound health themselves. She moved into a near-by newly opened hostel for disabled people—one that promoted and supported independent living. She eventually received Direct Payments—allowing her to employ her own personal assistants (PAs)—individuals with whom she could communicate and in whom she had confidence and trust. Helen grew to relish being responsible for every aspect of her lifestyle and welfare. She wrote of these years as follows: '*I had to decide for myself what time I would like help in getting up in the morning, what time I would like meals, what food to eat . . . It was both challenging and satisfying to take control of my existence, to decide for myself how I wanted to live. I am lucky enough to have a car which takes me sitting in my wheelchair, and this allows me to get out and about. I sit on various committees connected with disability. The aspect I value most about having a home of my own is the privacy, and not having the pressure of communal living*'.

Today: the need for End of life Support: Helen was diagnosed with terminal bowel cancer when she was 65, and knows that there are only a few months of life remaining. A specialist palliative care nurse assigned to her case has taken the trouble to learn how to communicate with Helen via the word board, and has established that Helen is desperately keen to stay in her own home and to die there . . .

Here are a few suggested answers, in brief, to the questions posed. Readers are asked to consider these, and to think through the other challenges and options involved:

1. What needs does Helen's position present to end of life support services?

Helen's 'needs' are certainly complex compared to cancer patients with no previous morbidity. A full assessment of her needs is required—an assessment that will consume extra time and resource—because continuous communication with Helen will be key, that is, meaningful communication that is not 'one-off' or tokenistic. Maintaining Helen's autonomy and meeting her preferences will demand much skill, patience, and respect on the part of the professionals and volunteers involved. Attitudes are of critical relevance here. The provision of appropriate specialist equipment, appliances and (possibly) medication is an obvious requirement in this case (both practically and ethically). Helen's right to make choices, and express her feelings and emotions, must be upheld throughout.

2. How can these best be met?

The quality of the training of staff cannot be underestimated in this case; minimalist 'tick the disability box' training will be entirely insufficient. Moreover, the policies that shape the services and practices available for the support of women and men in Helen's position must be up to the task if *equality* and *inclusion* is to be meaningful. More generally, the need for ongoing research and auditing to support *best practice* among professionals and services is implicated.

3. What other considerations come into play?

In Helen's case, close relatives are not involved—but family and legal guardians may well come into the scenario for other disabled people. If so, there is the danger that family members or guardians begin to make decisions *on behalf of* the disabled person at the end of life—particularly if this is because they *have always assumed the right to 'take charge' of the 'dependent'*. It would, of course, be entirely contrary to the disabled person's right to self-determination if professional staff and/or family members automatically collude in decision making about 'the care' of the 'unfortunate' disabled person. Clearly, this is extremely difficult territory for professionals who possess full knowledge of the rights of disabled people; their ability to *step carefully* will be in great demand.

References

Barnes, C. and Sheldon, A. (2010). Disability, politics and poverty in a majority world context. *Disability & Society*, **25**(7): 771–82.

Bickenbach, J. E., Chatterji, S., Badley, E. M., and Ustun, T. B. (1999). Models of disablement, universalism and the international classification of impairments, disabilities and handicaps. *Social Science and Medicine*, **48**: 1173–87.

Borsay, A. (2005). *Disability and Social Policy in Britain since 1750.* Basingstoke: Palgrave Macmillan.

Cabinet Office. (2004). *Improving the Life Chances of Disabled People.* London: Prime Minister's Strategy Unit.

Clark, D. and Seymour, J. (1999). *Reflections on Palliative Care.* Buckingham, UK: Open University Press.

Charlton, J. I. (1998). *Nothing about Us without Us: Disability, Oppression, and Empowerment.* Berkley: University of California Press.

Department of Health. (DH) (2007). *Cancer Reform Strategy.* London: DH.

Department of Health. (2008). *Better Care, Better Lives: Improving Outcomes and Experiences for Children, Young People and Their Families Living with Life-limiting and Life-threatening Conditions.* See www.dh.gov.uk/publications.

Emerson, E., Madden, R., Robertson, J., Graham, H., Hatton, C., and Llewellyn, G. (2009). *Intellectual and Physical Disability, Social Mobility, Social Exclusion & Health.* Submission to: *Strategic Review of Health Inequalities in England Post 2010* (Marmot Review). Lancaster University: CeDR Report 2.

Fisher, P. and Goodley, D. (2007). The linear medical model of disability: Mothers of disabled babies resist with counter-narratives. *Sociology of Health & Illness,* **29**(1): 66–81.

Friedlander, H. (1995). *The Origins of Nazi Genocide: from Euthanasia to the Final Solution.* Chapel Hill, NC: University of North Carolina Press.

Koffman, J. and Camps, M. (2008). No way in: Including disadvantaged population and patient groups at the end of life. In S. Payne, J. Seymour, and C. Ingleton (eds), *Palliative Care Nursing: Principles and Evidence for Practice,* 2nd edn. Maidenhead, UK: Open University Press, 362–82.

National Institute for Clinical Excellence (NICE). (2004). *Improving Supportive and Palliative Care for Adults with Cancer: The Manual.* London: NICE.

Marmot Review. (2010). *Fair Society, Healthy Lives: Strategic Review of Health Inequalities in England post-2010.* London: The Marmot Review.

Office of Disability Issues. (2010). www.officefordisability.gov.uk/. Accessed 16 Nov. 2010.

Officer, A. (2010). Research and policy working together to improve the lives of disabled people worldwide. Plenary Paper delivered to the Disability Studies Conference Sept. 2010, Lancaster University. Available at: www.lancs.ac.uk/cedr/.

Oliver, M. (1996). *Understanding Disability: From Theory to Practice.* London: Macmillan.

Oliver, M. and Barnes, C. (1998). *Disabled People and Social Policy: From Exclusion to Inclusion.* London: Longman.

Payne, S., Seymour, J., and Ingleton, C. (2008). *Palliative Care Nursing: Principles and Evidence for Practice,* 2nd edn. Maidenhead, UK: Open University Press.

People First. (2010). People First is an organisation run by and for people with learning difficulties in the UK. Accessed Nov. 2010: www.peoplefirstltd.com/.

Priestley, M. (ed.) (2001). *Disability and the Life Course: Global Perspectives.* Cambridge: Cambridge University Press.

Priestley, M. (2003). *Disability: A Life Course Approach.* Cambridge: Polity Press.

Roulstone, A. and Barnes, C. (eds) (2005). *Working Futures? Disabled People, Policy and Social Inclusion.* Bristol: The Policy Press.

Runswick-Cole, K. (2010). Living with dying and disablism: Death and disabled children. *Disability & Society,* **25**(7): 813–26.

Shakespeare, T. (1998). Choices and rights: Eugenics, genetics and disability equality. *Disability & Society*, **9**: 665–81.

Stein, G. L. (2008). Providing palliative care to people with intellectual disabilities: Services, staff knowledge, and challenges. *Journal of Palliative Medicine*, **11**(9): 1241–8.

Stein, G. L. and Kerwin, J. (2010). Disability perspectives on health care planning and decision-making. *Journal of Palliative Medicine*, **13**(9): 1059–64.

Thomas, C. and Curtis, P. (1997). Having a baby: Some disabled women's reproductive experiences. *Midwifery*, **13**: 202–9.

Thomas, C. (1999). *Female Forms: Experiencing Understanding Disability*. Buckingham, UK: Open University Press.

Thomas, C. (2007). *Sociologies of Disability and Illness Contested Ideas in Disability Studies and Medical Sociology*. Basingstoke: Palgrave Macmillan.

Thomas C., Morris S. M., and Clark, D. (2004). Place of death: Preferences among cancer patients and their carers. *Social Science and Medicine*, **58**(12): 2431–4.

Tomlinson, M., Swartz, L., Officer, A., Chan, K. Y., Rudan, I., and Saxena, S. (2009). Research priorities for health of people with disabilities: An expert opinion exercise. *The Lancet*, **374**(Nov.): 1857–62.

WHO Commission on Social Determinants of Health. (2008). *CSDH Final Report: Closing the Gap in a Generation: Health Equity Through Action on the Social Determinants of Health*. Geneva: World Health Organization.

WHO, ILO, and UNESCO. (2004). Joint Position P–CBR: *A Strategy for Rehabilitation, Equalization of Opportunities, Poverty Reduction and Social Inclusion of People with Disabilities*. www.who.int/disabilities/cbr/en/.

WHO. (2010). *Disabilities*. www.who.int/topics/disabilities/en/. Accessed Nov. 2010.

Part 2

Chapter 9

Death and dying in older people

Caroline Nicholson and Jo Hockley

Introduction and background

Chronological age is not directly tied to biological age, with many people remaining fit and active well into their nineties. However, the death and dying of those in very late old age challenge both individuals and society. These challenges are the focus of this chapter. This cohort of seniors, living in what is termed 'the Fourth Age', often contest the prevailing models of end of life care. The small but growing evidence demonstrates that dying older people are more likely to experience repeated hospital admissions, lack of preventive planning, social isolation, and economic hardship and are less likely to access specialist palliative care than their younger counterparts (Seymour et al., 2005). Indeed older people have been described as the 'disadvantaged dying' (Harris, 1990).

In this chapter we first consider the challenges of end of life care in late old age. We then introduce the concept of 'frailty' in older people and the importance of acknowledging dying in old age as a more natural event (McCue, 1995) than dying from cancer or other diseases earlier in the life course. We will explore the concept of 'natural dying' in the Fourth Age as both an opportunity and a challenge: an opportunity to maximize and learn from the capacity of those living and dying in late old age; a challenge to the current professionalization of death and dying within the developed world, where the focus is on medicalized and 'abnormal' death in the very frail older people. Finally, we look at care homes as a place where older people live and die. We set out the important role care homes now have in framing end of life care, the demands that beset them, and the aspiration that care homes could be significant in challenging society's taboo of death.

The challenges for end of life care in late old age

This Fourth Age, relating approximately to those people 85 years and older, is often associated with an inability of the mind and body to adapt, and an increase in cognitive and physical decline The threatened and actual losses associated with the Fourth Age lead to the assertion that 'living longer seems to be a major risk for human dignity' (Baltes and Smith, 2002: 3). In this chapter we argue that this construction of people living and dying in late old age fails to hold the complexity and possibility of individual and social growth. However, it is the prevailing lens through which death and dying in older age are viewed. The 'double bind' of being older and dying in Western culture is considered below.

Ageism and dying

Ageing is complex, and whilst considerable literature now relates positive and constructive attitudes to older people there is a balance between being over idealistic and nihilistic. Some argue the ambiguity and intricacies of late old age are not held well within culture, policy, and welfare (Biggs, 2005). Rather, there is a vacillation between 'successful ageing' as a time of extended consumerism, opportunity, and independence; and, 'unsuccessful' ageing as a time of increasing dependency and decreasing capacity. This stereotyping of people living in both Third and Fourth Age is imbued with ageism.

Ageism refers to the set of social relations that discriminates against older people and sets them apart as different as a result of an over-simplified and generalized definition and understanding of them. The setting apart of older dying people can be formulated as a social and individual defence against the anxiety and fear of getting older, of dependency, and of death. Such defences can lead to a denial of need, the diminishment of remaining capacity and fear of real engagement with older people (Davenhill, 2007).

There are important implications of ageism for dying—for older people themselves, those caring for them, and for wider society. Older people can feel a pressure to define themselves as 'less able' or 'fragile' and therefore withdraw from existing physical and social capacities; paradoxically this can lead to increased dependence (Nicholson, 2009). On the other hand, other older people may resist any form of help, preventative or secondary, for fear of being rendered helpless, and thus they potentially miss the appropriate level of support. Therefore older people are vulnerable to both over- and under-treatment at the end of life.

Defences against ageism and dying have organizational and societal consequences too. It has long been recognized that working with loss and dying has a profound effect on caregivers and their potential to remain appropriately involved (Menzies Lyth, 1988). However, perhaps because of ageist defences that can be hidden under the naturalness of dying in older age, carers (both formal and informal) of older people have received little emotional or organizational support. This is in sharp contrast to services for those caring for people dying from cancer (Froggatt, 2004). Rather, people dying in the Fourth Age (and their carers) are more likely to be socially set apart or sequestrated as their proximity to death is uncomfortable for society at large.

Increasing medicalization of people living in late old age

With the increasing opportunity for health care and treatment, there has been a growing medicalization of people living into late old age. Some argue that the intention to treat and not discriminate has led to a health care system that is 'ageist', in the sense that treatment often takes no account of age and the considerable loss of, and accommodation to, changing physical, intellectual or social ability in later life (McHugh, 2003). Thus acute services increasingly prioritize pace of care over complexity of need for older adults with the number of older people occupying a hospital bed rising to 65 per cent.

The development of palliative care was seen as a counter to the increasing medicalization of dying. However the growth of palliative care as a speciality and crucially the separation of care of older people from care of the dying has prioritized clinical intervention and the diagnosing of dying over the development of a wider public health model where dying is integrated into social life and viewed as a matter for families and communities (Kellehear, 2005). Currently in many UK trusts 'unexpected' deaths of frail older people are to be reported as an untoward incident. Some health care professionals find it difficult to acknowledge the old adage 'pneumonia is the old man's friend' and find it a considerable challenge to know when not to treat an older person (Seymour et al., 2005). However, disease must never outweigh the care of the patient and late old age must not be considered a disease that we can somehow cure.

The concept of frailty in late old age

Frailty and the experience of living in late old age are phrases often used inter-changeably. However there is an evolving endeavour among academics and clinicians to conceptualize and distinguish frailty from chronology. 'Frailty' has emerged as a key term in organizing services, including palliative care, for older people across the Western World (Grenier, 2007). With this has come an ever expanding literature on defining and managing frailty.

Whilst the concept of frailty is widely recognized, what constitutes frailty is not so clear. Frailty indices identify the deficits in health of an older person, be they symptoms, signs, diseases, disabilities or cellular and physiological abnormalities, on the grounds that the more deficits a person has, the more likely that person is to be frail. The debates about what indicators to use are ongoing, but the link between ageing, multiple morbidities, and frailty is clear. Sociological conceptions are critical of the dominance of health care practices that transform experience to problems. Their concern is that frailty is reduced to risk which diminishes people, objectifies need and rations services. Grenier's (2007) discussion of the etymology of frailty progresses this idea. She notes that frailty is defined in the *Oxford English Dictionary* as a fault and infirmity with both physical and moral dimensions. Using a Foucauldian analysis, she goes on to extrapolate that frailty is a practice which divides (or classifies) in order to provide or restrict care. Frailty has been defined as a dying trajectory (Lynn and Adamson, 2003) associated with multiplicity of loss and an increasingly dwindling, downward trajectory towards dying.

Nicholson (2009) argues that frailty in later life is a state of 'in-betweeness' in which people experience *the loss* of some connections whilst trying to *sustain* others and perhaps *create* new ones. Crucially, the struggle in old age to *hold together* loss and continuity is contained within the wider context of the gradation into death. In becoming frail, people begin to inhabit the space between living and dying. Nicholson argues that it is this space between life and death that is not held well within current policy and practice. Rather, 'dying work' is held within a professional palliative care ideology and seen as something to be sequestrated, not part of the normal development of the life course. Her study suggests that holding together loss and creativity is the ordinary, but none the less remarkable, experience of frail older people. Creativity within psycho-social interpretations of frailty is linked to the capacity to mourn.

In frailty, it is necessary to mourn losses and ultimately your own life before it is possible to invest part of yourself in people and things that will outlive you. For frail older people the presence of people to engage with stories, recognize and value the daily rituals that anchor experience and facilitate creative connections is vital to retain capacity, quality of life and the natural development into dying. However, Nicholson (2009) suggests that this engagement can be compromised by loneliness, ageism, and the present over-emphasis in health and social systems on assessing need through physical functionality. Whilst necessary attention is being given to diagnosing the point of dying in older people, the uncertain dying trajectory of many people in their fourth age requires a greater engagement with both living and dying through everyday interactions.

How does frailty intersect with terminal care, palliative care and end of life care?

End of life care is a term that is currently being used to denote the holistic needs and support of a person nearing the end of their life (DOH, 2008). However, end of life was originally used within the literature on frail older people to encompass the wider range of diseases that older people die from and encompasses the care required to support people living and dying over time. (Fisher et al., 2000).

Whilst frailty and end of life care are not synonymous, both concepts try to capture something of the challenges and experience over time within a life long-lived. Within end of life care there is an encouragement and facilitation of an open approach to the awareness of dying. However, despite the aspirations of end of life care, most literature on older dying people focuses on the defined terminal phase. Yet it is often the accumulation of losses that become significant for older frail people. These accumulated losses, termed 'living bereavement' (Katz, 2003), have significant impact for families and staff alike.

The imperative to address end of life care for older people is a pressing political and social issue. In England 66.8 per cent of deaths occur in people 75 years and above, with 1 in 6 of these deaths occurring in people aged 90 years or over (NEoLCIN, 2010). The social connections in which older people are embedded constitute a major source of personal well-being and a principal resource for end of life care in later life. However social networks and the care they provide is increasingly precarious with children moving away from the family, transient neighbourhoods and social care whose configuration often militates against consistency and time to work 'with' rather than 'on' frail older people.

Whilst the hospice movement has grown considerably, societal attitudes towards death and dying remain largely unchallenged. However, we argue that the broadening of services for the dying in late old age into care homes and an emphasis on the natural development into dying could be a lever for change. Allowing a considered natural death, instead of an over-treated dying (i.e. the often futile attempt to re-start a heart), brings a dignity to dying in very late old age. We argue this dignity is often compromised by an emphasis on medical treatment and the concerns over risk and litigation.

The Care Home context

It is estimated that in the UK 53.6 per cent of people of the Fourth Age live in care homes (Brown Wilson and Davies, 2009). The concept of the 'nursing home' dates back to the fourth century. The historical texts of the Byzantine period (324 to 1453 AD) highlight the human-orientated behaviour embraced by the Byzantine emperors, the church, and individuals; they showed great interest in older people, and founded many welfare institutions. The nursing homes for the old were called 'Gerocomeia'. In the seventeenth century, workhouses/poorhouses were being built in both England and the Netherlands.

During the 1980s across the USA, Australia, Canada, and the UK, governments began to be more proactive about the care of frail older people in late old age. In the UK long-stay geriatric wards in acute hospitals were closed in favour of privately run care homes. The modern care home has now become a multi-billion-dollar business across the developed world and even in developing countries. In the UK there is now three times the number of private care home beds compared to beds within the NHS (Badger et al., 2009). The funding of such care is hugely diverse across the developed world with different funding policies. In the USA 'not for profit' care home organizations have developed as a result of the ethical pressure of making a profit when many older people because of mental and physical frailty would find it difficult to evaluate the quality of care given. Dementia is one of the most common diagnoses amongst care home residents (Small et al., 2006). This is mirrored across Canada, the USA, Australia, and the UK, where two-thirds of residents are likely to have a degree of dementia (Hockley, 2010).

Care homes are currently one of the most regulated industries across the developed world. Whilst there has been some justification for this, at the same time a huge amount of paperwork has to be completed, keeping the limited number of qualified nurses away from day-to-day care. In the 1990s in the UK, regulators insisted on an overall staffing level of 1:5 (nursing) and 1:6 (residential). Now care home managers are expected to provide the necessary staffing levels according to dependency; in reality, the staffing levels have not changed despite increasing dependency creating a huge pressure when it comes to end of life care. Care home regulation has been seen to present a narrow focus on dying and death (Froggatt, 2007), with standards on death and dying only being monitored every few years. In Scotland, care home standards (SPPC, 2006) are written with a wider focus ensuring aspects of end of life care are appropriately monitored.

Embracing care homes as a place where older people die

Around the developed world, care homes are now taking on the role of end of life care with increasing numbers of deaths occurring in the care home. In the USA, 43 per cent of individuals who reach 65 years of age will spend time in a nursing home (Reynolds et al., 2002) with 25 per cent of all USA deaths occurring in long-term care; this figure is predicted to rise to 1 in 2 deaths by 2020 . In the UK and Australia on average 1 in 5 people over the age of 65 years die in care homes (DOH, 2008). The majority of these UK deaths occur within the 4,300 nursing care homes and this is where most development in end of life care has taken place.

There is a danger that because the hospice movement is accepted as an example of good practice in death and dying, that such a model be replicated for the care of frail older people dying in care homes. However, hospices/specialist palliative care units and care homes have very different contexts. The hospice movement developed its expertise from the care of people dying from cancer. In care homes, there are generally fewer than 10 per cent of cancer patients—cancer is not often a disease of the Fourth Age. A more typical person requiring palliative care in care homes is likely to be an 86-year-old woman with congestive cardiac failure, diabetes, osteoarthritis, and mild dementia.

It is important therefore for a collaborative model to develop between specialist palliative care services and staff in care homes or long-term facilities (Chenoweth and Kilstoff, 2002; Hockley, 2006) rather than imposing a hospice model with little consideration of the different types of disease. This is not to say that staff in care homes cannot learn a considerable amount from hospice and specialist palliative care services, but specialist palliative care professionals need to be cognizant of the different diagnoses and indeed the expertise that staff in care homes already have.

The End of Life Care Strategy in the UK (DOH, 2008) highlights the importance of care homes in the development of high quality end of life care. However, when developing practice in care homes it is important to consider not only the appropriateness of the evidence to be introduced but also the context and the level of facilitation (Froggatt, 2002). It is unlikely that the implementation of evidence-based tools into care homes will be successful unless there is 'high facilitation' because of the generally acknowledged 'weak' culture (Hockley et al., 2010).

Quality end of life care in care homes

Despite a considerable percentage of the population of countries in the developed world dying in care homes/long term facilities, research highlights that there are challenges in developing appropriate end of life care. Staff shortages, poor recruitment and retention, reliance on untrained staff, lack of medical input, isolation from training, lack of a learning culture, poor knowledge of symptom control, and a closed communication culture are some of the challenges that need to be overcome (Hockley, 2006; Ersek and Wilson, 2003). However, where the organizational emphasis is on ensuring a good quality of life with an 'openness' to recognizing death as a significant event rather than striving to keep alive, and where there are good working relationships with the wider multidisciplinary team and a keen interest to develop knowledge, the care home can be a place that equals the care given by staff in any hospice. Brazil et al. (2004) highlight six themes that contribute to high-quality end of life care (see Box 1).

Symptoms such as depression, pain, constipation, and anorexia are considerable problems for frail older people. The importance of maintaining quality through appropriate assessment and management underpins good care. However, the assessment of symptoms has in the past been the remit of the doctor and with some nursing homes having inadequate medical input this can be a problem (Glendinning et al., 2002). In the Netherlands, medical services and allied health professionals such as physiotherapists have always been part of the overall nursing home structure giving greater support and multi-disciplinary working.

In the UK, strategies for improving end of life care in generalist settings such as care homes have focused around the implementation of systems or tools such as the Gold Standards Framework for Care Homes, Advance Care Planning and the adapted Liverpool Care Pathway (DOH, 2008). Systems such as the above that help staff open up discussion in relation to death and dying in a sensitive and appropriate manner are very important in order to counteract the dominant culture of restorative and

> ## Box 1 Themes for quality end of life care in care homes [data from Brazil, 2004]
>
> - Responding to residents' needs
> - Creating a home-like environment
> - Support for families
> - Providing quality care processes
> - Recognizing death as a significant event
> - Having sufficient institutional resources.

rehabilitative care. However, tools are only as good as the person using them. Indeed, without appropriate training, role modelling, and staff support, tools on their own can do more damage than good. Where such tools have been implemented with adherence to proper implementation and facilitation there have been encouraging results (Hockley et al., 2005; Hockley et al., 2010). These include not only improved outcomes but also additional benefits such as: improved teamwork, more meaningful communication, increased critical awareness which influences practice and creates improved openness in relation to death and dying (see Box 2).

High quality end of life care is not just about those people who are dying. It is about the relationship that these people have with other frail older people who they know, their families and those who are there to support them both socially and clinically.

Conclusion

It has been said many times that the hallmark of a society is the way it provides for its weakest and most vulnerable. In this chapter we have stressed the importance and potential of a natural death in very late old age, both for individuals and society at

> ## Box 2 Extract highlighting 'open communication' around death and dying
>
> . . . 'I went along following D and the undertaker down the corridor, walking behind the coffin . . . and all the doors of the residents rooms were open. And the ones that could were sitting near their door; they had wheeled themselves to the door. And when I got to the reception, the night staff that were coming on duty were standing there and all the day staff who had looked after him that he was very fond of, were there. . . . that was really, really lovely, actually. And D said to me, "Oh, I never asked them to do that . . . I did go into all the residents telling them that [your Dad] had passed away—'do you want us to close the door?' And everyone said 'No!'". That was nice–that was really nice . . .'
> [NHG, Rel 2—Hockley et al., 2004].

large. Clearly there are many challenges. However, we argue that there is a growing evidence base on end of life care for older people and that care homes are vital in providing this. It is important that both clinical and social support are available if older people are not to be marginalized and society as a whole remain in denial about death. Ongoing conversations are required, which include older people themselves, about the best way to celebrate and allow for the end of a life long lived. We offer this chapter as part of this dialogue.

Resources

◆ 'My Home Life' is a national movement aimed at improving the quality of life for people living, dying, visiting, and working in care homes for older people. See http://myhomelifemovement.org.

◆ 'National End of Life Care Intelligence Network—Dementia' is a network which holds useful, up-to-date information on statistics and other reports in relation to end of life care. See www.endoflifecare-intelligence.org.uk/data_sources/dementia.aspx.

References

Badger, F., Clifford, C., Hewison, A., and Thomas, K. (2009). An evaluation of the implementation of a programme to improved end-of-life care in nursing homes. *Palliative Medicine*, **23**: 502–11.

Baltes, P. and Smith, J. (2002). New frontiers in the future of ageing: From successful ageing of the young old to the dilemmas of the Fourth Age. Key note lecture at the Valencia Forum, Valencia, Spain, April 1–4, www.mpib-berlin.mpg.de/en/forschung/lip/Baltes-Smith.pdf.

Biggs, S. (2005). Beyond appearances: Perspectives on identity in later life and some implications for method. *Journal of Gerontology: Social Sciences*, **69b**(3): S118–27.

Brazil, K., McAiney, C., Caron-O'Brien, M., Kelley, M. L., O'Krafka, P., and Sturdy-Smith, C. (2004). Quality end of life care in long-term care facilities: Service provider's perspective. *Journal of Palliative Care*, **20**(2): 85–92.

Brown Wilson, C. and Davies, S. (2009). Developing relationships in long term care environments: The contribution of staff. *Journal of Clinical Nursing*, **18**: 1746–55.

Chenoweth, L. and Kilstoff, K. (2002). Organisational and structural reform in aged care organisations: Empowerment towards a change process. *Journal of Nursing Management*, **10**: 235–44.

Davenhill, R. (ed.) (2007). *Looking Into Later Life: A Psychoanalytic Approach to Depression, Dementia and Old Age*. London: Karnac.

DOH. (2008). *End of Life Care Strategy*. London: Department of Health.

Ersek, M. and Wilson, S. A. (2003). The challenges and opportunities in providing end-of-life care in nursing homes. *Journal of Palliative Medicine*, **6**(1): 45–57.

Fisher, R., Ross, M., and MacLean, M. (2000). *A Guide to End of Life Care for Seniors*. Ottawa: University of Toronto and University of Ottawa.

Froggatt, K. (2007). The 'regulated death': A documentary analysis of the regulation and inspection of dying and death in English care homes for older people. *Ageing & Society*, **27**: 233–47.

Glendinning, C., Jacobs, S., Alborz, A., and Hann, M. (2002). A survey of access to medical services in nursing and residential homes in England. *British Journal of General Practice*, **52**: 545–8.

Grenier, A. (2007). Constructions of frailty in the English language: Care practice and the lived experience. *Ageing and Society*, **27**(3): 425–45.

Harris, L. (1990). Continuing care: The disadvantaged dying. *Nursing Times*, **86**(22): 26–9.

Hockley, J., Watson, J., and Dewar, B. (2004). Developing quality end of life care in eight independent nursing homes through the implementation of an integrated care pathway for the last days of life. Unpublished full report.

Hockley, J. M., Dewar, B., and Watson, J. (2005). Promoting end-of-life care in nursing homes using an 'integrated care pathway for the last days of life'. *Journal of Research in Nursing*, **10**(2): 135–52.

Hockley, J. (2006). Developing high quality end of life care in nursing homes: An action research study. Unpublished PhD thesis, University of Edinburgh.

Hockley, J., Watson, J., Oxenham, D., and Murray, S. (2010). The integrated implementation of two end-of-life care tools in nursing Care homes in the UK: An in-depth evaluation. *Palliative Medicine* (in press).

Katz, J. (2003). Managing dying residents. In J. Katz and S. Peace (eds), *End of Life in Care Homes: A Palliative Care Approach*. Oxford: Oxford University, 59–74.

Kellehear, A. (2005). *Compassionate Cities: Public Health and End-of-life Care*. Oxfordshire: Routledge.

Lynn, J. and Adamson, D. (2003). Living well at the end of life: Adapting health care to serious chronic illness in old age. Santa Monica: RAND Health.

McCue, J. (1995). The naturalness of dying. *JAMA*, **273**(13): 1039–43.

McHugh, K. (2003). Three faces of ageism: Society, image and place. *Ageing and Society*, **23**: 165–85.

Menzies Lyth, I. (1987/8). The psychological welfare of children making long stays in hospital: An experience in the art of the possible. In I. Menzies Lyth (ed.), Containing Anxiety in Institutions: Selected Essays, vol. 1. London: Free Association Books, 130–207.

NEoLCIN. (2010). Deaths in Older Adults in England. National end of Life Care Intelligence. Accessed 10 Oct. 2010: www.endoflifecare-intelligence.org.uk.

Nicholson, C. (2009). Holding it together: A psycho-social exploration of frailty in Old Age. Unpublished PhD dissertation. London: City University.

Reynolds, K., Henderson, M., Schulman, A., and Hanson, L. C. (2002). Needs of the Dying in Nursing Homes. *Journal of Palliative Medicine*, **5**(6): 895–901.

Seymour, J., Witherspoon, R., Gott, M., Ross, H., Payne, S., and Owen, T. (2005). *End of Life Care: Promoting Comfort, Choice and Well Being for Older People*. London: Policy Press.

Small, N., Froggatt., K., and Downes, M. (2007). Living and dying with dementia: Dialogues about palliative care. Oxford: Oxford University Press.

Chapter 10

Vulnerable adults and families

Malcolm Payne

An important social difference exists between people who are vulnerable to harm from adverse events and those who are resilient. Vulnerable people must expend more energy and resources in protecting themselves against misfortune and social and health care agencies may have to expend effort and resources in protecting them. Dying people are more vulnerable than most others, leading to an enhanced responsibility for services to protect them. Advanced illness or disability may reduce their capacity to protect themselves and increase susceptibility to adversity, and approaching the end of life may increase pressures on them or their families.

Are palliative care services responsible for protecting vulnerable adults and families? Everyone living in social groups has informal responsibility for safeguarding others, particularly vulnerable people. The first line of protection is therefore the families and communities surrounding vulnerable people. Most people accept responsibility for the safety of children because they may not have the maturity or development to protect themselves. However, adulthood confers individual autonomy: what is the point at which we decide to intervene with an autonomous adult because of concerns about their vulnerability and safety?

Legislation and administrative procedures exist to surround people with a safe environment. Mandelstam (2009) summarizes the following areas of British law on the subject; this analysis suggests the range of areas to consider:

- the policy and legal responsibilities of health, social care and emergency services for responding to the needs of vulnerable adults.
- the regulation of care provision.
- arrangements for dealing with mental incapacity that may mean that adults cannot make their own decisions about their lives.
- arrangements for protecting the safety of the environment, for example housing and local community safety, of older people.
- protecting older people from physical and sexual harm and abuse.
- protecting older people from financial abuse, not only by family members but by commercial and financial service providers.

This legal provision for health and safety is controversial, because the argument for autonomous personal responsibility for self-protection has to be balanced with the duty of care held by professionals to vulnerable people.

The legislative basis of the role of social and health care services focuses on safeguarding older people and other vulnerable adults from abuse, exploitation, and harm.

The duty varies in different jurisdictions. The autonomy argument means that in many legal systems no direct intervention can be made, for example to remove an abuser or shift a victim to a safe place. However, much abuse is a criminal offence and legal action may be possible, which may be a warning to perpetrators of abuse, or may protect the client. In many states of the US and in Scotland, legislation makes specific provision for protective services. Elsewhere, and in England and Wales, safeguarding is among the responsibilities of official social services agencies. Scotland is an example of a jurisdiction where intervention is authorized. The Adult Support and Protection (Scotland) Act 2007 requires local social services authorities to promote cooperation between agencies and to make inquiries if allegations come to their attention. It also provides for legal orders to require assessments of situations that are identified to be carried out, to remove someone who is at risk from a particular situation or to ban an abuser from being present in the home of an abused person. A review of the procedures and guidance in England in 2008–9 has not led to similar developments.

The legal and administrative bases for understanding vulnerability and abuse also vary. The UK model is founded in human rights. The official guidance (Department of Health/Home Office, 2000: 9) defines abuse as 'a violation of an individual's human and civil rights by any other person or persons'. No single term is used for elder abuse in state legislation across the US, and descriptive terms such as abandonment, mental anguish, exploitation, neglect, self-neglect, and sexual abuse are the most often used (Daly and Jogerst, 2001).

Further protection is often accorded to people who have insufficient mental capacity to protect themselves, for example through learning disabilities, mental illness, or dementia. In the UK, as an example, this includes provision for people to take over decision-making on their behalves and protection through the 'deprivation of liberty safeguards' against arbitrary restraint of freedom of action (Department of Constitutional Affairs, 2007).

Abuse, neglect, and self-neglect

Evidence of abuse and neglect of vulnerable adults has increased since its recognition in the 1980s. The initial concern was about abuse and neglect arising from poor-quality care in institutions providing care for older people and people with long-term conditions, such as learning disabilities and mental illness. Evidence of abuse and neglect by informal and paid carers in people's own homes emerged. More recently, a distinction has been made between abuse and neglect arising from carer stress and domestic violence affecting vulnerable adults (Bergeron, 2001).

The picture of abuse is consistent across the world. Both patients and carers may be perpetrators of abuse: an Australian study (Livermore et al., 2001) estimated that about 75% of elder abuse was of the person being cared for and 25% of the carer. Saveman and Sandvide's (2001) Swedish study of GPs' experience of abuse found that risk situations commonly involved patients with dementia, carers with problems of their own or who felt angry about the burden of caring, or paid carers who were unable to meet the needs of an older person. Payne's (2008a) audit of safeguarding cases at St Christopher's Hospice, London, identified pre-existing mental illness in the family and alcohol and drug use as factors underlying some abuse of palliative care patients. Goergan's (2001) study of German nursing homes found that 59% of staff report physical or verbal aggression by residents during the previous two months, 79% of staff indicate having abused or neglected a resident at least once during that period; 66% witnessed victimizations of residents by colleagues. Staff perceptions associated staff abuse with work stress and poor working conditions as well as the psychological predisposition of perpetrators.

Self-neglect is a persistent inattention to maintaining personal hygiene and a safe environment, persistent refusal of appropriate services and endangering health and safety by failing to take reasonable protective actions, such as effective wound care or fire prevention safeguards (Pavlou and Lachs, 2008). This behaviour builds up over time and it is unclear whether it is associated with deteriorating cognitive functioning among older people or whether the origins are mainly social; both factors may be relevant. Choi et al. (2009) found in a Texas study that self-neglect was associated mainly with poverty, poor health care and poor family support rather than mental incapacity. Lauder et al.'s (2009) British qualitative study suggests that self-neglect is not only associated with older people, but with long-standing chaotic lifestyles, due to mental illness or drug abuse. Intervening is difficult because older people's autonomy prevents professionals from being engaged, and self-neglect may also isolate the older person, so that the problems are not reported. They may also be reported inappropriately as presenting housing problems or public health hazards.

Prevalence of abuse and neglect

A systematic study of prevalence studies across the world (Cooper et al., 2008) found that 6% of the older population, 25% of vulnerable adults, and a third of family caregivers report being involved in significant abuse, but only 1–2% of this is reported officially. However, if they are directly asked, older people and their caregivers are prepared to report it, so it is important to ask. A UK prevalence study (O'Keefe et al., 2007) found 2.6% of people aged 66 and over, living in private households, reported mistreatment involving a family member, close friend or care worker during the past year. This rose to 4% including people such as neighbours and others not in a trust relationship. Since most dying people are older people, these percentages suggest the minimum likely levels of abuse in palliative care caseloads. Yan and Tang's (2001) Hong Kong study found prevalence rates of 2% for physical abuse and 20.8% for verbal abuse among elders participating in the study. Abused elders, as compared with non-abused elders, scored significantly higher on psychological distress and were significantly more dependent on their caregivers.

The qualitative UK prevalence study (Mowlem et al., 2007) identifies barriers in reporting abuse such as low self-confidence, bereavement, physical frailty, and not taking mistreatment seriously enough. Other barriers were fear of the consequences, such as alienating carers, and uncertainty about where to report abuse and whether doing so would bring benefits. Incentives for disclosing abuse were fears for personal safety and encouragement from others. This suggests that practitioners can help people to disclose and deal with abuse.

Approaches to intervention

People may disclose abuse when they want services to do something about it. Barriers and incentives to patients making disclosures, discussed above, also affect staff who are unaccustomed to dealing with abuse issues (Payne, 2005). Practitioners therefore need to be confident in their knowledge of reporting and investigation procedures to reassure patients and colleagues about confidentiality and respect for patients' preferences. Practitioners and agencies likely to find safeguarding issues in their work should therefore be engaged with and able to influence local networks of protective services, so that policy and processes are appropriate for their user group.

In addition to preventive social and health care services supporting vulnerable populations, a range of direct safeguarding interventions is required, but there is little research to demonstrate what combination of strategies achieve effective outcomes. Social work approaches are the main intervention, since social work agencies are usually responsible for investigation and service provision with vulnerable adults. Social work builds on counselling and educational approaches and also engages directly in family mediation and service provision (Payne, 2007, 2008b). By building supportive relationships with vulnerable people, with family members and informal caregivers, social work practitioners identify different priorities among the people involved and mediate between them to achieve improvements in behaviour and interpersonal relationships. Social workers also assess preferences and needs of patients, family members and caregivers to identify and plan appropriate services to meet needs that cannot be met from within the family and community.

A counselling approach involves working with a patient or family member to help them identify personal, practical or psychological difficulties and develop strategies for reducing or removing the social consequences of those difficulties. Educational interventions may be needed to assist caregivers develop appropriate skills, for example in manual handling or anger management, or patients with assertiveness. A rights-focused approach aims to assess types of abuse and reasons for its taking place, identify risk factors in victims' situations and clarify how they may assert their rights when such situations arise again. In Cripps's (2001) Australian study this was completely effective in 50%, partly helped in 34%, and led to no change in 16% of cases.

Safeguarding services

Fallon (2006) describes New Zealand provision, identifying four elements of a safeguarding service:

- ◆ Local services to support vulnerable people and respond to difficult or risky situations.
- ◆ Professional health and social care interventions to help and protect individuals experiencing abuse and neglect.
- ◆ Advisory group support for professionals engaged in this difficult work and local coordination of services.
- ◆ National policy development and coordination.

The first element is prevention. If general social and health care services are wide-ranging and sufficient, carers and vulnerable people can get early support for difficulties. Effective advance or anticipatory care planning (Payne, 2011: 2) can help people to avoid extempore solutions to complex problems. Completion, before the onset of frailty, illness or mental incapacity of advance decisions is important. Examples are wills, proxies to take over decision-making in case of incapacity, such as, in the UK, lasting powers of attorney both for legal and financial and personal welfare affairs, or in the US, appointment of proxies, to take decisions for people with mental incapacity. 'Advance decisions' or directives provide legally enforceable statements of the patient's wishes not to receive particular treatments (Csikai and Chaitin, 2006).

The main elements of protection are: immediate safety for the vulnerable person, documenting abusive or neglectful behaviour in preparation for any investigation, reporting abuse to the appropriate agency, and cooperating in long-term plans for protection of the vulnerable person, according to their preferences (Gray-Vickrey, 2001).

Investigation of allegations of or concerns about abuse starts from contacts with all professionals and informal and community caregivers involved, to see the extent to which concerns are shared. Signs of abuse picked up by individuals, when coordinated by a case conference or similar meeting, may suggest a pattern of problems. Agencies may then agree strategies for protection. These often involve training and support for informal caregivers, increased surveillance by coordinating different professionals' visits to the vulnerable person's home and alternative or additional care such as day care. Occasionally, particular dangers, such as inappropriate visitors, may need to be removed or supervised.

Palliative care interventions

Palliative care services are rarely in the front line of managing safeguarding. However, abuse of older people is often connected with carer stress. Most dying people are in this age group and need additional informal care; moreover their increasing ill-health increases their vulnerability, so that accustomed patterns of family relationships, such as robust shouting matches as a form of communication, may need to change. Care homes, hospital wards and even hospice in-patient units where poorly trained and supervised staff are the main contact with dying patients also present risks of institutional abuse through paid carers' stress.

Palliative care teams are not exempt from poor reporting rates of abuse and neglect. One American study (Liao et al., 2009) found a statistically significant difference between adult protection and palliative care professionals in the likelihood of identifying and reporting cases of abuse; 30% of palliative care professionals had suspected but not reported abuse within the previous five years. Among palliative care professionals, 11% had ethical concerns and 63% concerns about the practical consequences of reporting abuse; 90% would report abuse that they witnessed, but only 63% would report abuse reported by the patient. Only 37% correctly identified the appropriate agency for reporting concerns. Policy at St Christopher's Hospice, therefore, focused on ensuring that all practitioners should be *alert* to the possibility that abuse might occur, *aware* of procedures to report abuse and protect victims, and *active* in taking action (Payne, 2008a).

Because, in many jurisdictions, social work agencies take the primary role in investigating safeguarding concerns, social work palliative care team members should play an important role in safeguarding. Christ et al. (2010) argue that social workers' roles in developing family caregiver and support in palliative care teams places them in a good position to take leadership in safeguarding aspects of palliative care interventions. A counselling model of practice is inappropriate, because active intervention in family relationships is required for safeguarding.

Since the palliative care aim in safeguarding practice is a positive outcome for patients in the dying process, a useful social work objective is to attempt to achieve security for a victim of abuse. Security may be both physical and emotional and has a number of different aspects in practice:

- Physical security, for example avoiding unwanted change in carers. violence, or fear of it.

- Legal security, for example feeling that the law and administrative procedures protect them rather than hindering them in achieving their tasks in the last few weeks of life.

- Self-security, being respected and valued by others (Payne, 2011: 8).

Conclusion

Vulnerability to abuse and neglect is increased for dying people compared with the general population. However, abuse, neglect, and self-neglect are poorly identified and reported in all social and health care settings, including palliative care. Carer stress and domestic violence are important factors in abuse and neglect, and self-neglect occurs because of poor social and health care resources and chaotic lifestyles in all age groups, rather than mental incapacity mainly among older people.

Both victims and health care staff may lack confidence that there will be positive outcomes from reporting and knowledge of how to report abuse and neglect. Preventive strategies through engagement with national and local coordination and through interventions with families are required to identify perpetrators and safeguard vulnerable people from abuse, neglect and self-neglect. Counselling, educational, social work, and rights-based interventions are available but robust effectiveness research is not available. Much therefore requires to be done to achieve a good death for dying people who experience abuse and neglect.

Resources

- The Social Care Institute for Excellence provides a number of authoritative documents covering all client groups, including reviews of research and practice guidance; many are regularly updated: http://www.scie.org.uk/.
- The UK prevalence and qualitative research on elder abuse in the UK is available at: http://www.dh.gov.uk/en/Publicationsandstatistics/Publications/Publications-PolicyAndGuidance/DH_078333.

♦ The best source of up-to-date information in the UK is the local authority for the area covered, and there is often comprehensive documentation of national as well as local policy. An internet search for (name of the local authority).gov.uk is likely to bring the best results; if your authority is weak a good alternative is to look at the materials produced by another authority.

References

Bergeron, L. R. (2001). An elder abuse case study: caregiver stress or domestic violence? You decide. *J Geront Soc Wk*, **34**(4): 47–63.

Choi, N. G., Kim, J., and Asseff, J. (2009). Self-neglect and neglect of vulnerable older adults: Reexamination of etiology. *J Geront Soc Wk*, **52**(2): 171–87.

Christ, G., Stein, G. L., Blacker, S., and Kayser, K. (2010). Social work leadership in palliative care: Developing family and caregiver support intervention models. *J Pain Symptom Manag*, **39**(2): 319–20.

Cooper, C., Selwood, A., and Livingston, G. (2008). The prevalence of elder abuse and neglect: A systematic review. *Age & Ageing*, **37**(2): 151–60.

Cripps, D. (2001). Rights focused advocacy and elder abuse. *Australasian Journal on Ageing*, **20**(1): 17–22.

Csikai, E. and Chaitin, E. (2006). *Ethics in End-of-life Decisions in Social Work Practice*. Chicago: Lyceum.

Daly, J.M. and Jogerst, G. (2001). Statute definitions of elder abuse. *J Elder Abuse Neglect*, **13**(4): 39–57.

Department of Constitutional Affairs. (2007). *Mental Capacity Act 2007: Code of Practice*. London: The Stationery Office.

Department of Health/Home Office. (2000). *No Secrets: Guidance on Developing and Implementing Multi-agency Policies and Procedures to Protect Vulnerable Adults from Abuse*. London: Department of Health.

Fallon, P. (2006). *Elder Abuse and/or Neglect*. Wellington, NZ: Ministry of Social Development.

Goergen, T. (2001). Stress, conflict, elder abuse and neglect in German nursing homes: A pilot study among professional caregivers. *Journal of Elder Abuse & Neglect*, **13**(1): 1–26.

Gray-Vickrey, P. (2001). Protecting the older adult. *Nurs Manag*, **32**(10): 36–40.

Lauder, W., Roxbrugh, M., Harris, J., and Law, J. (2009). Developing self-neglect theory: Analysis of related and atypical cases of people identified as self-neglecting. *J Psych Ment Health Nurs*, **16**: 447–54.

Liao, S., Jayawardena, K. M., Bufalini, E., and Wiglesworth, A. (2009). Elder mistreatment reporting: Differences in the threshold of reporting between hospice and palliative care professionals and adult protective service. *Palliat Med*, **12**(1): 64–70.

Livermore, P., Bunt, R., and Biscan, K. (2001). Elder abuse among clients and carers referred to the Central Coast ACAT: A descriptive analysis. *Aust J Ageing*, **20**(1): 41–7.

Mandelstam, M. (2009). *Safeguarding Vulnerable Adults and the Law*. London: Jessica Kingsley.

Mowlam, A., Tennant, R., Dixon, J., and McCreadie, C. (2007). *UK Study of Abuse and Neglect of Older People: Qualitative Findings*. London: National Centre for Social Research.

O'Keeffe, M., Hills, A., Doyle, M., McCreadie, C., Scholes, S., Constantine, R., et al. (2007). *UK Study of Abuse and Neglect of Older People: Prevalence: Survey Report*. London: National Centre for Social Research.

Pavlou, M. and Lachs, M. S. (2008). Self-neglect in older adults: A primer for clinicians. *J Gen Intern Med*, **23**(11): 1841–6.

Payne, M. (2005). Adult protection cases in a hospice: an audit. *J Adult Protect*, **7**(2): 4–12.

Payne, M. (2007). The role of social work in end of life care. *End of Life Care*, **1**(1): 69–73.

Payne, M. (2008a). Safeguarding adults at end of life: Audit and case analysis in a palliative care setting. *J Soc Wk End-of-Life Pall Care*, **3**(4): 31–46.

Payne, M. (2008b). Safeguarding of vulnerable adults at the end of life. *End of Life Care*, **2**(1): 42–6.

Payne, M. (2011). *Humanistic Social Work: Core Principles in Practice*. Chicago: Lyceum.

Saveman, B.-I. and Sandvide, Å. (2001). Swedish general practitioners' awareness of elderly patients at risk of or actually suffering from elder abuse. *Scand J Caring Sci*, **15**: 244–9.

Yan, E. and Tang, C. S. (2001). Prevalence and psychological impact of Chinese elder abuse. *J Interpers Violence*, **16**(11): 1158–74.

Chapter 11

Dying as a teenager or young person

Anne Grinyer

Introduction

Simon's Story

When Simon, an Australian aged 18, was diagnosed with terminal cancer, he decided that never having previously left Australia he would spend the remainder of his life travelling: he left university and persuaded two of his fellow students to accompany him to England. The impact on his parents of 'allowing' him the independence to undertake this adventure was profound; he forbade them from accompanying him or following him. His parents never saw him alive again—a younger child would be unable to make such a decision and an older adult might not feel the need to.

When his condition deteriorated significantly Simon's parents were contacted by the hospice in London who were offering Simon support and a 'hotel' service. They immediately set off to London but heard during a stopover in Singapore that he had died. While deeply distressing for his parents, in some ways Simon's death might be considered a 'good death'; he died doing what he wanted to do, surrounded by professionals who understood his life stage and supported him with age-appropriate care. Simon trusted that the hospice could supply anything he needed; his mother said that at one point when he and his friends were going out they wanted a taxi and had no number to call; Simon said 'Ring the hospice—they'll know'. After Simon's death his mother spoke of the sensitivity with which the staff had laid him out, respecting his youth culture. The age-appropriate nature of the care can best be summed up by his mother Helen as follows:

> They'd dressed him in his favourite black T-shirt and jeans. It was hard to get used to the dyed hair he'd had done just before he left. It was his last chance for a bit of teenage rebellion—black dye with purple highlights. (It sounds worse than it looked.) The nurses said the purple came off on their hands.

Background

Teenagers and young adults (TYAs) facing the end of life are socially different, they are neither children nor fully fledged adults, and their transitional life stage can cause great challenges to both their families and their health care providers (Grinyer, 2002). They can fall between care settings in a way that can be distressing for all concerned.

TYAs aged 16–24 receive end of life care in a variety of care settings including adult and paediatric hospital wards, age-specific cancer units, children's, adult, and adolescent hospices, and they are also supported to die at home. The fact that end of life care is provided in such a diverse range of settings, most of which are not designed specifically to meet the needs of the age group, suggests a variety of experience that may be contingent on local provision. Yet as Craig (2006) argues, the palliative care needs of young people in this age group are significantly different from those of adults and children in physical, social, psychological, and emotional terms.

While many of the examples drawn on in this chapter are UK based, it is important to recognize that geographical and cultural differences can affect requirements. For example, in Australia, Journeys (2005) acknowledge that the needs of those from rural or remote areas, indigenous families and culturally diverse backgrounds need consideration as their needs will differ; Goldman et al. (2006: 557) recognize that in poorly resourced countries the concept of palliative care is 'just not "awake"', nevertheless, they document countries such as Romania as having adopted a number of effective palliative care programmes for young people, but recognize that there are still barriers to those working in a country such as Romania which has only 'pockets of awareness' (562).

There have been a number of studies, particularly from the field of oncology, which demonstrate that when serious illness occurs during adolescence and young adulthood particular challenges are experienced by the patient, their families, and their care providers (Albritton et al., 2003; Grinyer, 2002; Kelly, 2008). As Kelly and Gibson (2008) argue, it is a phase of emotional and social development frequently characterized as 'problematic' and marked by acts of separation and rebellion.

There can be a lack of 'fit' for TYAs who, when treated in a paediatric setting, will be cared for by staff who have chosen to work with children while those in an adult setting will be used to more mature adults, however, caring for adolescents can be demanding as their behaviours can present challenges for which staff may be unprepared. They may have anxieties about their emerging sexuality, fertility, relationships, education, and their appearance all of which are normal causes of concern for the age group and which are exacerbated by illness (Grinyer, 2007). In addition, the setting of care in paediatric and adult services can be experienced as alienating by some TYAs. They may be irritated by being treated alongside young children in a child-orientated environment and can be intimidated by an adult setting where they may be in a bed next to a person in their seventies or eighties. Thus this life stage, falling as it does between paediatric and adult settings, has been identified as requiring an age-appropriate approach to care (Apter, 2001; Arbuckle et al., 2005; Grinyer, 2007).

TYAs have been recognized as requiring well-planned transition and age-appropriate care, but many of the studies focus on long-term or acute care; yet when the care relates to end of life the difficulties can be exacerbated. The studies on end of life care and place of death for this age group tend to be statistical and do not tell us much about the experience or how choices have been made (Montel, 2009; Feudtner et al., 2003; Higginson et al., 2003). One of the few qualitative studies to focus on end of life care for adolescents was conducted in France and suggests that the palliative care of adolescents and young adults needs considerable improvement if it is to meet their needs at the end of life more effectively (Montel, 2009: 35).

The teenagers' and young adults' perspective

The majority of TYAs cared for in children's hospices have been born with or have developed chronic or life-limiting illness in early childhood. For those who have been using the children's service since their infancy there can be an increasing awareness that being surrounded by small children and crying babies in a setting designed to appeal to much younger children is inappropriate. While children's hospices can continue to care for young people up to 30 years old, for the adolescent patient this may become an alienating environment.

The expressed need for a more age-appropriate care setting by the long-term users of a children's hospice indicates that familiarity is not enough for them to remain satisfied with an environment they have outgrown. Nancy, whose daughter Tess at 26 had used the hospice services since she was 14, said that Tess would have valued a more 'grown up' setting and 'doesn't like the children crying and screaming'. This suggests a child-orientated culture where older users can begin to feel out of place and parents may also feel marginalized. If this is problematic for the young people to whom the care setting is very familiar, the situation for the TYA who is suddenly diagnosed with a life-threatening condition may be even more challenging. One children's hospice with a higher than usual number of referrals of young people with cancer had attempted to make their environment appealing by providing a 'teenaged' room. Although some TYAs agreed to investigate the possibility of care here they did not agree to become inpatients. The reasons are summed up by the head of clinical services as follows:

> One of the challenges really is that although we try and make the environment suitable for all age groups, as you walk in you probably notice it . . . leans towards the younger age group, with the number of fluffy toys and things around . . . one young person of 16 referred to our service had quite an aggressive tumour and was obviously coming towards the end of their life . . . came to see the service here . . . and she felt that this environment wasn't right for her . . . [despite the fact that] one of our rooms is very specifically teenagery.

It is unusual for an adult hospice to be asked to accept a young person with a chronic life-limiting condition who will be more likely to stay on for care in a children's setting. However, young adults diagnosed with acute and life-threatening illness—particularly cancer, in which adult hospices in the UK tend to specialize—may seek end of life care in such a setting. Yet even for those young people at the older end of the age range, the likelihood of patients in adult hospices being perceived as 'elderly' can make the setting unacceptable. Ryan, at 22, was offered a bed in an adult hospice for his end of life care, and while the facilities and environment were excellent and the staff friendly, he and his wife Bianca, aged 20, felt out of place. Bianca said:

> I don't feel that they really understood us as a young couple. And in my head a hospice was somewhere old people went to die and . . . it was lovely and the rooms they showed us were really wonderful . . . and the nurses were really nice, but . . . no one was his age there.

A similar account was offered by Ellen's mother Ann, who told me that Ellen, who died at home aged 23, had been offered care in an adult hospice, but much too soon. In the event she had another three years to live—this indicates how difficult it can be to predict accurately when end of life plans should be made. One of Ellen's health care professionals, Sarah, said: 'She was deserted in the middle of a busy, adult ward and could see people who were really poorly . . . she'd stood in the middle of the ward and sobbed . . . she found the whole experience a nightmare.' This put her off to such an extent that she refused to consider care there at any future stage.

For one young man, Stuart, who died at home just before his eighteenth birthday, the issue was that he was treated like a child by the paediatric community nurses, as his mother Joan said: 'unfortunately, because they are community nurses . . . and they [are] used to seeing . . . little children, they treated him as if he was about six'. This attitude caused Stuart great annoyance and resulted in his resentment of the nurses' 'invasion' of his home. Thus for home-based care, too, consideration of an age-appropriate approach should be central if TYAs are not to feel a lack of fit with the service.

Perhaps one of the issues most challenging to both parents and their young adult sons and daughters is giving them intimate care. For a TYA who is sexually mature the invasiveness of nursing or medical procedures can be distressing, but the embarrassment can be exacerbated if parents are called upon to wash, clean, and toilet their adult children. Brenda, whose son Miles (23) was cared for at home, said the following:

> Often he had soiled himself during the night and woken up demoralized. With a young child, a parent can make light of such things but in our case we were always 'treading on hot coals'. (Grinyer, 2002: 27)

This infringement of privacy can be discomforting to all concerned, particularly when coupled with the potential threat to their sexuality and sexual identity and the impact on their appearance. All these issues are of central concern in this age group; thus to be faced with the physical manifestations of the illness and its treatment can be experienced as particularly distressing. The situation can be equally upsetting for young people who have lived their whole lives with chronic conditions. Although they may be more used to receiving intimate care from their parents, when as adolescents they become aware of changes in their bodies, increased sensitivity is needed in order that they maintain their dignity. Again this is a life stage issue which if recognized and dealt with sensitively by professionals can help to ameliorate the situation.

Parents' and families' perspective

Many of the young people in this age group will still be dependent financially on their parents. Even if they had been living independently they will probably return to their family of origin as the infrastructure of adolescent and young adult life is unlikely to be able to support end of life care. This can result in resentment against the enforced dependence and in challenging behaviours; it can also impact upon siblings and throw the household into turmoil.

While most TYAs who receive care at home do so in their parents' homes, there are exceptions which may make the situation even more complex; for example, if the young person is married—as was the case with Bianca and Ryan, who had no choice but to move in with Ryan's mother. Bianca spoke of the struggle she had with Ryan's mother over the 'control' of Ryan's care. As Bianca said: 'I felt she became very competitive towards the end about who did this for him and who did that'; and of course Ryan's end of life care was taking place on his mother's territory and in his childhood bedroom, the symbolism of which threatened to render Bianca powerless. In a variation of this situation Pat, the mother of Sara, told me that she was insistent that Sara wanted to 'die alone with her husband [Brad] and her cat'. Pat spoke of the struggle she had to accept that Brad was Sara's primary carer; at one point Pat said Sara had sat them all down and told them: 'I can no longer be in the middle of this. I cannot be your mediator. You have to talk to each other.'

Professionals' perspective

In addition to the adult hospice environment being unappealing to a young person, the staff may be unused to TYAs' propensity to 'pad around in the early hours of the morning', while their fierce and sometimes challenging manifestations of independence and control which can be swiftly followed by needy and childlike behaviour can be difficult to manage. A balance also has to be struck between allowing the teenagers to 'be teenagers' and the needs of the older patients whose patterns, behaviours, and preferences are very different. The staff may also be unused to caring for a patient who is 'dying out of time'. Young people often have very difficult deaths; although it may seem paradoxical, their bodies are quite strong and 'don't just gently fade away'.

Recognizing the lack of fit, some hospices have gone beyond the provision of an adolescent room and have built an adolescent wing, annexe, or separate facility for young adults up to 40 years old. These age-specific hospices provide an ideal transition for the long-term users of the children's hospices and bridge the gap between paediatric and adult services for those young people who have chronic life-limiting conditions. But what about the young adult diagnosed in their adolescence with an acute illness? The concern for those planning such a service has been that despite an age-appropriate care setting, the environment would not appeal to young adults with acute illness. Much work on supporting a TYA emphasizes the importance to them of maintaining 'normality' which is key to the age group, yet they may not identify with the young adult hospice users who, while close in age, are not similar in any other way. Nevertheless, in two young adult hospices a model of good practice appears to have been developed which is fostered by a philosophy of specialized care that focuses predominantly on the age group, maximizing the similarities between the different users while attempting to minimize the differences.

It seems that if handled with sensitivity and skill such a setting can be appealing—and indeed enjoyable—yet such age-specific facilities are still unavailable to most teenagers and young adults as they are so few and far between. However, even if the environment can be made appealing to teenagers and young adults there is an additional implication for the training of staff in both paediatric and adolescent hospices. Liz, Head of Care at a hospice for young adults, pointed out that skills around very complex symptom control and pain management are essential but may not be familiar.

Similarly additional skills are needed in children's hospices where there may be little experience of cancer and where staff may also be unused to the demands of a dying TYA.

Multi-professional clinical care may address some of these issues. This is a highly valued approach in both paediatric and adult oncology and is arguably of even greater significance in the care of TYAs but professionals will need to be both willing and able to cross the paediatric/adult divide. An effective multi-professional team can ensure continuity of care, provide a comprehensive view of the patient, contribute a range of skills, and offer mutual support and education (Morgan, 2005: 259–60).

A team-based approach that includes professionals expert in the psycho-social dimensions may assist with the difficulties in communication. TYAs occupy the territory between childhood and adulthood; this can make it difficult for professionals to know how to share information and manage decision-making. Parents may try to protect their sons and daughters from full awareness and this can create ethical dilemmas for professionals who value an open awareness context. A dedicated meeting at an early stage with both the TYA and the parents can circumvent later problems if the management of information and the flow of communication can be agreed in advance. This may mean that the TYA is told first then the information is repeated in a meeting with the whole family when decisions can be made jointly. However, some TYAs may prefer their parents to be told and for them to pass on the information. Levels of maturity at this age are only loosely related to chronological age so individual assessments of each family need to be made.

The implications for provision

It can be seen that for this transitional age group there is a lack of fit in many settings of end of life care—so what can be done to meet their needs? Hospices for adolescents and young adults are expensive to develop, few and far between, and while they may be very apt for young people with chronic life-limiting conditions, at present they do not always offer an acceptable environment to young people with acute terminal illness. The option of building specialist hospice units for young adults with cancer is not feasible financially. So it seems that if appropriate provision is to be made for young people with both chronic and acute conditions it needs to be based on current services.

There are a number of measures that might address the challenge. Firstly, shared care between hospitals and hospices could work in both directions, so the hospice staff can help to deliver end of life care in a hospital setting. Alternatively staff from the age-specific care centres can offer support and advice to hospice staff after they have discharged a patient to their care. For such shared care to work requires good relationships being established in advance between the hospital and hospice so that boundary issues do not arise. One way of achieving this might be the development of training packages that can be implemented if and when a young person in the age group requires support and care at the end of life.

Given such constraints, it seems that the best way in which to approach end of life care for this age group is to adopt a philosophy of care that borrows from that which underpins specialist adolescent care in the acute setting. If it is possible to get the philosophy right, the physical setting can usually be adapted without too much difficulty. It is important that those with complex, chronic, and life-limiting conditions also have their status as adolescents recognized and catered for, and this may require some input from children's hospices in forward planning. As Robinson and Jackson (1999: 69) say: 'Local residential units, offering a degree of privacy and autonomy with on-call personal assistance, could also be a stepping stone to supported/independent living'.

A limitation of this chapter is that it has not addressed the needs of young people who are at additional social disadvantage such as those who are refugees or asylum seekers. However it is likely that the lack of easy 'fit' experienced by the TYAs who are not socially disadvantaged is likely to be exacerbated for those who have further problems of language, status, and social marginalization. Thus the needs of those with additional social differences and complex family lives must also be recognized.

Conclusion

The provision of age-appropriate end of life care to adolescents and young adults is an issue now very much on the agenda. The particular needs of the age group have been recognized in policy documents and measures are being taken to meet those needs. Individual hospices are responding to the needs of their adolescent and young adult users both chronic and acute and are taking steps to ensure that the care setting is age-appropriate. Even if resources are limited, if the philosophy that underpins age-appropriate care can be implemented across the range of hospice provision and coupled with training packages, shared care, and early planning for transition, this will make a significant contribution to meeting the needs of the age group. The example of Simon, thousands of miles from his home in Australia, cared for by staff at an adult hospice who fully respected his age, life stage, and need to live the remainder of his life as a teenager, demonstrates the fact that a philosophy of care can be implemented across a range of settings if there is motivation, understanding, and sensitivity.

Resources

+ Association of Children's Palliative Care. (2007). *The Transition Care Pathway.* Bristol: ACT; www.endoflifecareforadults.nhs.uk/eolc/files/ACT-Transition_care_pathway_Apr2007.pdf.
+ Goldman, A., Hain, R., and Liben, S. (eds). (2006). *Oxford Textbook of Palliative Care for Children.* Oxford: Oxford University Press.

References

Albritton, K. and Bleyer, W. A. (2003). The management of cancer in the older adolescent. *European Journal of Cancer*, **39**(18): 2584–99.

Apter, T. (2001). *The Myth of Maturity: What Teenagers Need From Parents to Become Adults.* New York: W. W. Norton.

Arbuckle, J., Cotton, R., Eden, T. O. B., Jones, R., and Leonard, R. (2005). Who should care for young people with cancer? In T. O. B. Eden, R. D. Barr, A. Bleyer, and M. Whiteson (eds), *Cancer and the Adolescent.* Oxford: Blackwell, 231–40.

Craig, F. (2006). Adolescents and young adults. In A. Goldman, R. Hain, and S. Liben (eds), *Oxford Textbook of Palliative Care for Children.* Oxford: Oxford University Press, 108–18.

Department of Health. (2008). *Better Care: Better Lives–Improving Outcomes and Experiences for Children, Young People and Their Families Living With Life-Limiting and Life-Threatening Conditions.* Retrieved from: www.dh.gov.uk/en/Publicationsandstatistics/Publications/PublicationsPolicyAndGuidance/DH_083106. Accessed 14 Feb. 2010.

EAPC. (2009). *Palliative Care for Infants, Children and Young People.* Retrieved from: www.eapcnet.org/download/forTaskforces/Paediatric/PC-FACT.pdf. Accessed 14 Feb. 2010.

Feudtner, C., DiGiuseppe, D. L., and Neff, J. M. (2003). Hospital care for children and young adults in the last year of life: A population-based study. *BMC Medicine*, 1: 3.

Goldman, A., Southall, D., Lenton, S., and Eaton, N. (2006). International aspects. In A. Goldman, R. Hain, and S. Liben (eds), *Oxford Textbook of Palliative Care for Children*, Oxford: Oxford University Press:557573.

Grinyer, A. (2002). *Cancer in Young Adults: Through Parents' Eyes.* Buckingham, UK: Open University Press.

Grinyer, A. (2007). *Young People Living with Cancer: Implications for Policy and Practice.* Buckingham, UK: Open University Press.

Higginson, I. and Thompson, M. (2003). Children and young people who die from cancer: Epidemiology and place of death in England (1995–9). *British Medical Journal*, 327: 478–9.

Journeys—Palliative Care for Children and Teenagers. (2005). Palliative care in Australia. Retrieved from: www.palliativecare.org.au/Default.aspx?tabid=1120. Accessed 6 April 2010.

Kelly, D. (2008). The physical and emotional impact of cancer in adolescents and young adults. In D. Kelly and F. Gibson (eds), *Cancer Care for Adolescents and Young Adults.* Oxford: Blackwell, 23–43.

Kelly, D. and Gibson, F. (2008). Introduction. In D. Kelly and F. Gibson (eds), *Cancer Care for Adolescents and Young Adults.* Oxford: Blackwell.

Montel, S., Laurence, V., Copel, L., Pacquement, H., and Flahault, C. (2009). Place of death of adolescents and young adults with cancer: First study in a French population. *Palliative and Supportive Care*, 7: 27–35.

Morgan, S. (2005). Managing professional relationships across the services. In T. O. B. Eden, R. D. Barr, A. Bleyer, and M. Whiteson (eds), *Cancer and the Adolescent.* Oxford: Blackwell, 259–69.

Robinson, C. and Jackson, P. (1999). *Children's Hospices: A Lifeline for Families.* London: National Children's Bureau.

Chapter 12

People with intellectual disabilities

Irene Tuffrey-Wijne

Introduction

An estimated 1–3 per cent of the world's population have intellectual disabilities (Mash et al., 2004). They are among the most vulnerable and disadvantaged groups in society. England has an ageing population: by 2021, the number of people with intellectual disabilities over the age of 50 is expected to have increased by 53 per cent (Emerson et al., 2008). Such increased longevity leads to a rising incidence of life-limiting illnesses such as cancer (Hogg et al., 2008) or dementia (Visser et al., 1997).

Until as recently as the 1980s, many people with intellectual disabilities in Western society who did not stay with their families lived and died in segregated institutions. Their health care was of little concern for mainstream providers. In this new millennium, the requirement to provide equitable palliative care to increasing numbers of people with intellectual disabilities at the end of life (many of whom now live more independent and integrated lives in society) is a considerable challenge for primary care providers, hospitals and hospices.

The poor quality of health care people with intellectual disabilities receive has been well documented. In the UK a range of reports have highlighted consistently the poor quality of care for people with intellectual disabilities in both primary and acute secondary health care (Disability Rights Commission, 2006; MENCAP, 2007). A report into access to health care for people with intellectual disabilities concluded that they experienced discrimination, abuse, and neglect across the range of health services (Michael, 2008).

How, then, can we best meet the palliative care needs of this group? Are these needs different from those of the rest of the population, and if so, how? There is a growing body of literature around the particular issues facing people with intellectual disabilities at the end of life, and those that support and care for them (for example, McLaughlin et al., 2009; Read, 2006; Tuffrey-Wijne, 2009; Wagemans et al., 2010), although empirical data remain scarce.

In this chapter, the term 'intellectual disability' is used, as this appears to be recognized and acceptable in most countries. In the UK the term 'learning disability' is often used. There are three aspects to the definition of intellectual disability: (1) significant limitations in intellectual functioning, together with (2) significant limitations in adaptive behaviour as expressed in conceptual, social, and practical skills, which (3) originates before the age of 18 (Schalock et al., 2010).

Case study

Pete Carpenter was 66 years old and had severe intellectual disabilities. His speech was limited to short sentences. When his parents died 25 years ago, he moved into a staffed residential home in London. The memories of his younger years, filled with steam trains and jazz music, always remained important; his family were a crucial part of that. His closest relative was his sister who visited twice a year.

Pete's diagnosis of lung cancer was made after months of coughing and weight loss, at which stage his prognosis was only a few months. As soon as the sad news was broken to the managers of his home, a meeting was called with his key carers to discuss ways of managing Pete's illness and ensuring that the last months of his life were as good as they could be. This included referrals to the district nurses and the local hospice palliative care team.

There were some major concerns. Pete was as yet unaware of his diagnosis, and although his carers agreed that he should be told in order to avoid collusion, nobody knew how best to do this. After much debate, Pete was given the bad news by a general practitioner, with a trusted carer present. He never asked any questions, and did not show any signs of distress; in fact he seemed to accept his deteriorating health with grace.

His carers were keen to keep him at home, but there were concerns about the inadequate physical layout of the house, which was not designed to support people with increasing health care needs. Pete's bedroom was upstairs, and during the last few weeks of his life, he was too weak to manage the stairs. There was a discussion about the feasibility of Pete sleeping in the downstairs living room, but this had unacceptable consequences for the two other residents, who were deeply worried about Pete. In the end, Pete's deterioration was so fast that no difficult decisions about where he should be cared for needed to be taken. His bed was moved downstairs temporarily, and he died there when both other residents were away for the weekend; this was considered lucky by many. What would have happened to Pete if he had needed a longer period of intensive caring at home? One of his fellow residents was always very generous and accom-modating, but confided in her day centre manager: 'It's OK for you, you go home at the end of the day. I have to sit there and watch it.'

A palliative care nurse from the local hospice visited the home to give Pete's carers advice and support. It was difficult for her to assess Pete's needs and symptoms, because he often misunder-stood her questions and did not clearly indicate his pain. (Whenever Pete had to go into hospital for further tests, there were similar problems; hospital staff were often insensitive to his needs, and could not work out what he was saying.) The palliative care nurse probably underestimated the amount of support needed by his carers, who were frightened by Pete's illness and worried about his impending death, and about how they were going to cope. In the UK, carers in intel-lectual disability services are usually untrained, often young, and mostly very inexperienced in death and dying. Pete was given morphine to control his pain, but the carers were anxious about this. They were not sure when they could give him extra analgesia, or what they should do when Pete was too weak to swallow the medication. Pete rarely complained of pain; he had experi-enced severe pain in childhood and had somehow learned not to show it.

The days leading up to Pete's death were very difficult for his carers. They realized that he was getting very weak, and they did not have enough practical support to manage his care. Pete him-self was calm and simply slipped into unconsciousness fairly suddenly. The carers did not realize that he was dying, and rang an ambulance, panic-stricken about his sudden deterioration. The ambulance crew arrived after Pete died, tried to resuscitate him and took his body to hospital. The home manager was deeply distressed by this, and a year later he still blamed himself for ring-ing for that ambulance, rather than letting Pete die and stay peacefully at home.

Pete's sister did not visit him during his illness. She found it too distressing, and wanted to remember him as a healthy man. Pete's care staff didn't realize how important Pete and his sister were for each other—a crucial part of their past, of themselves; their sibling was part of who they were. Two years after Pete's death she still missed him deeply. 'He was a special brother,' she said. 'I am always thinking about him, and talk about him a lot with my husband. He was my only brother. People don't understand that.'

Pete Carpenter's story forms part of a research study and is more fully described in *Living with Learning Disabilities, Dying with Cancer* (Tuffrey-Wijne, 2010).

Issues in the provision of palliative care for people with intellectual disabilities

From Pete's story, several challenges emerge, many of which have also been highlighted in the growing body of literature in this field.

Late diagnosis

By the time Pete's cancer was diagnosed, the disease was already too advanced for treatment. Published case reports show that late presentation of the illness can be a result of problems with identifying symptoms and diagnostic overshadowing (where symptoms are attributed to the intellectual disability itself, rather than an underlying physical illness), resulting in advanced disease and severe symptomatology (Tuffrey-Wijne et al., 2007). Preventable illness may be missed as a result of inadequate screening.

Communication problems

Communication issues are often quoted as a major barrier to care. Many health care professionals do not feel confident in their ability to communicate with people with intellectual disabilities and to understand their communication, particularly if verbal ability is lacking (Tuffrey-Wijne et al., 2008). In Pete's case, his communication difficulties caused concerns around information giving, understanding, capacity and consent, symptom assessment, and general assessment of need.

Capacity and consent

The law around capacity and consent will vary between countries, but the underlying principle that people with intellectual disabilities have a right to be involved as much as possible in decisions around their treatment and care is an important one. In Pete's case, several health care professionals made assumptions about his (in)ability to understand his situation.

Disclosure

Existing models for breaking bad news seem to be inadequate for people with intellectual disabilities, and often people with intellectual disabilities are simply not helped to understand their diagnosis or prognosis (McEnhill, 2008). Pete's carers were unusual in their insistence to support his understanding, confidence or professional guidance in this area was lacking. The author is currently researching a workable and appropriate framework for breaking bad news to people with intellectual disabilities, with results expected in 2011.

Family

The family bonds of people with intellectual disabilities are hugely important. The effect of family relationships is often underestimated, particularly if the person has moved out of the family home at an early age, perhaps into residential care. Like Pete's sister, many family members experience strong feelings of distress and guilt when someone is suffering from a life-limiting illness. Paid caregivers do not always appreciate the importance of these bonds, and may resent the emergence of relatives who may not have been a regular presence in the person's life. Sensitive professional support is needed to help both the daily care givers and the family members.

Needs of care staff

In the UK, intellectual disability staff are among the poorest paid and poorest trained professionals in the country, and have low status. Many are young and inexperienced in issues around death and dying, leading to significant fear. Linda McEnhill writes: 'Despite this, many learning disability workers confront daily significant loss, emotional pain, and physical challenge . . . they receive little in the way of clinical supervision and due to budget restraints are not eligible for the vast range of educational opportunities' (McEnhill, 2004: 111). When a client is terminally ill, the challenges facing such staff are enormous. Outside professionals (including specialist palliative care staff) may well underestimate the support and information needs of intellectual disability care staff. Many experienced palliative care staff did their medical, nursing or social work training several decades ago in the era of segregation, and have little experience with people with intellectual disabilities. They may lack confidence in their ability to support this client group, thinking (or perhaps hoping) that intellectual disability staff already have the expertise to cope with end of life care issues.

Bereavement and loss

Most palliative care professionals will meet people with intellectual disabilities who are the dying patient's relative. The emotional life of people with intellectual disabilities has only been given thought in the past two decades. Many people with intellectual disabilities have experienced a huge amount of loss in their lives. They are at high risk of experiencing complex grief. Possible problems include the concept and understanding of death; difficult attachment originating in early childhood; and environmental issues, including a lack of recognition of the person's grief and a lack of social support (Blackman, 2003). Warmth and understanding are important; in some cases, skilled professional support is needed to help someone in their bereavement.

People with intellectual disabilities living in residential care settings can be greatly affected by the death of a fellow resident, and their bereavement needs must not be overlooked. Some care homes experience the death of a number of residents within a relatively short time frame, which can be very hard not only for the staff but also for the residents. The impact on other residents of someone dying in a care home must be carefully considered, and support provided. Openness and clarity about what is happening, and involvement of the residents in the care of their dying friend—as well as opportunities to remember and grieve together after the death—can be very helpful.

Resilience

It is important not to lose sight of the strengths of people with intellectual disabilities. Pete amazed those around him by his apparently calm acceptance of his situation (despite a longstanding fear of death) and his insistence to 'keep going' with his favourite activities, even when he was very ill. In our study of 13 people with intellectual disabilities who had cancer, including Pete Carpenter, people's resilience seemed to have a number of features. They were 'experienced sufferers': many had led difficult lives that seemed to have prepared them in some way for the challenges of debilitating illness. They were expert at 'living in the moment': most had an outlook of realism and practicality. One woman with a fungating breast cancer may not have understood the intricacies of cancer, but she agreed that a 'messy breast' was no good, so it was better if it came off (mastectomy). They were experienced at being cared for, and maybe more accepting than the general population of the loss of control that comes with serious illness. They gained huge comfort from having one or two committed carers. And, like Pete, many simply 'kept going' with what they liked doing, doggedly holding on to familiar routines and activities.

International context

The vast majority of the literature around palliative care and intellectual disabilities comes from the UK. Some of the issues highlighted in Pete Carpenter's case may well be unique to the English context. It has already been mentioned that differences in the law around capacity and consent will affect palliative care provision.

Some of the particular challenges in this area will be universal, such as communication difficulties, presentation of the illness and assessment of symptoms. The need to anticipate changing health care needs and make adequate resources available is also likely to affect services everywhere. One USA survey found that intellectual disability service providers were unprepared for the effects of an ageing population (Botsford, 2004).

However, there may also be particular problems inherent in the way each country has organized both intellectual disability services and palliative care services. Most researchers conclude that good collaboration between these two services is key to successful end of life support, but to what extent practitioners can act on this clearly depends on what services are available, and how they work.

In some countries, such as the Netherlands, the intellectual disability workforce includes many trained nurses and is therefore better prepared than their English counterparts to cope with physical deterioration in their client group. The risk here may be that intellectual disability staff may not invite specialist support, particularly if their service is centralized or perhaps institutionalized. A survey of Dutch intellectual disability providers found that collaboration with palliative care specialists was often lacking (Speet et al., 2006).

The reader is advised to keep their local realities in mind with regards to the following practice guidance.

Practice guidance for palliative care professionals

Many of these issues may appear complex and almost impossible to overcome, but relatively simple measures can often make a real difference.

- Find out as much as you can about the person's life story. Ask people to bring in photographs. Listen carefully to whatever the person communicates to you. Talk to family, carers and close friends.

- Introduce yourself each time you meet. Always address the person directly. Be prepared to allow some extra time.

- Use all possible communication methods to help the person understand what is happening, and to enable informed consent. This could include simple and repeated explanations, the use of pictures, or demonstration (e.g. showing someone a clinic or equipment beforehand).

- Follow the legal framework for capacity and consent in your country.

- If the person lacks capacity, set up a case review or best interest meeting, and involve family and friends and relevant professionals, as well as an independent mental capacity advocate if appropriate and available. The role of an advocate is to represent the interests of the individual, particularly when there are no relatives or friends to do so. How best interest decisions are taken, and exactly who is involved, will depend on the law of the country.

- Collaborate with other health care professionals, intellectual disability staff and families. Make contact with the intellectual disability professionals if they are available in your area.

- Assess pain and symptom control, as the person may not complain of pain openly. Regnard et al. (2007) developed the 'DisDAT', a tool for assessing distress in people with severe communication difficulties (see also www.disdat.co.uk/).

- Make reasonable adjustments to ensure that people with intellectual disabilities have the same access to end of life care pathways as other people.

- Allow the person's existing routines to continue if possible. Try to turn necessary medical procedures into a new routine. Try to have the same nurses look after the person each time.

- Offer support to the person's families and carers.

- Remember to involve, include, and support fellow residents, both before and after the death.

- Recognize the person's strengths, and use them.

Conclusion

With commitment, forward planning, collaboration, and above all a positive attitude, the provision of palliative and end of life care for people with intellectual disabilities can be a positive and inspiring experience for those involved. Palliative care professionals and other professionals in health and social care settings have much to contribute. Situations involving people with intellectual disabilities at the end of life are often complex, and a wide range of expertise is needed. No single professional paid carer or family member has all the skills and knowledge, but together they can form a strong team offering positive support.

Resources

- ◆ Tuffrey-Wijne, I. (2010). *Living with Learning Disabilities, Dying with Cancer: Thirteen Personal Stories* (London: Jessica Kingsley). This book, written in non-scientific language, gives the full findings of an ethnographic study of people with learning disabilities who died of cancer, including a full account of the stories of the participants (such as Pete Carpenter). It provides insight and advice for a range of professionals and care givers.
- ◆ *Books Beyond Words Series*, edited by S. Hollins, published by RCPsych Publications/St George's, University of London; www.rcpsych.ac.uk/publications/booksbeyondwords.aspx. A series of picture books for adults with learning disabilities, explaining difficult issues without the use of words. Titles include books on cancer and screening, going to hospital, and dying.
- ◆ Palliative Care for People with Learning Disabilities (PCPLD) Network, which brings together practitioners from a range of backgrounds to share information, experiences, and resources. The website has a Resources Page, see: www.pcpld.org.

References

Blackman, N. (2003). *Loss and Learning Disability*. London: Worth Publishing.

Botsford, A. (2004). Status of end of life care in organizations providing services for older people with a developmental disability. *American Journal on Mental Retardation*, **109**: 421–28.

Disability Rights Commission. (2006). *Equal Treatment: Closing the Gap—A Formal Investigation into Physical Health Inequalities Experienced by People with Learning Disabilities and/or Mental Health Problems*. London: Disability Rights Commission.

Emerson, E. and Hatton, C. (2008). *People with Learning Disabilities in England*. Lancaster: Centre for Disability Research.

Hogg, J. and Tuffrey-Wijne, I. (2008). Cancer and intellectual disabilities: A review of some key contextual issues. *Journal of Applied Research in Intellectual Disabilities*, **21**: 509–18.

Mash, E. and Wolfe, D. (2004). *Abnormal Child Psychology*. Belmont, CA: Thomson Wadsworth.

McEnhill, L. (2004). Disability. In D. Oliviere and B. Monroe (eds), *Death, Dying and Social Differences*. Oxford: Oxford University Press, 97–118.

McEnhill, L. (2008). Breaking bad news of cancer to people with learning disabilities. *British Journal of Learning Disabilities*, **36**: 157–64.

McLaughlin, D., Barr, O., and McIlfatrick, S. (2009). Delivering palliative care to those with a learning disability. *European Journal of Palliative Care*, **16**: 302–5.

MENCAP. (2007). *Death by Indifference*. London: Mencap.

Michael, J. (2008) *Healthcare for All: Report of the Independent Inquiry into Access to Healthcare for People with Learning Disabilities*. London: Aldrick Press.

Read, S. (2006). *Palliative Care for People with Learning Disabilities*. London: Quay Books.

Regnard, C., Reynolds, J., Watson, B., Matthews, D., Gibson, L., and Clarke, C. (2007). Understanding distress in people with severe communication difficulties: Developing and assessing the Disability Distress Assessment Tool (DisDAT). *Journal of Intellectual Disability Research*, **51**: 277–92.

Schalock, R., Borthwick-Duffy, S., Bradley, V., et al. (2010). *Intellectual Disability: Definition, Classification, and System of Supports*. Washington, DC: AAIDD.

Speet, M., Francke, A., Courtens, A., and Curfs, L. (2006). *Zorg rondom het levenseinde van mensen met een verstandelijke beperking: een inventariserend onderzoek* ('End-of-life care for people with intellectual disabilities: A scoping study'). Utrecht: Nivel.

Tuffrey-Wijne, I. (2009). The preferred place of care for people who are dying. *Learning Disability Practice*, **1**: 16–21.

Tuffrey-Wijne, I. (2010). *Living with Learning Disabilities, Dying with Cancer: Thirteen Personal Stories*. London: Jessica Kingsley.

Tuffrey-Wijne, I., Hogg, J., and Curfs, L. (2007). End-of-life and palliative care for people with intellectual disabilities who have cancer or other life-limiting illness: A review of the literature and available resources. *Journal of Applied Research in Intellectual Disability*, **20**: 331–44.

Tuffrey-Wijne, I. and McEnhill, L. (2008). Communication difficulties and intellectual disability in end-of-life care. *International Journal of Palliative Nursing*, **14**: 192–7.

Visser, F., Aldenkamp, A., van Huffelen, A., Kuilman, M., Overweg, J., and van Wijk, J. (1997). Prospective study of the prevalence of Alzheimer-type dementia in institutionalized individuals with Down Syndrome. *American Journal on Mental Retardation*, **101**: 400–12.

Wagemans, A., van Schrojenstein Lantman-de Valk, H., Tuffrey-Wijne, I., Widdershoven, G., and Curfs, L. (2010). End of life decisions: An important theme in the care for people with intellectual disabilities. *Journal of Intellectual Disability Research*, **54**: 516–24.

Chapter 13

People with mental health needs

Annabel Price and Max Henderson

Introduction

Exclusion of individuals with mental health problems from social roles and opportunities preceded the identification of their difficulties as 'mental health' in origin. Ideas of possession or 'animality', in which the madman was 'not sick' but in fact 'protected . . . from whatever might be fragile, precarious or sickly in man', underlay 'treatment' with forced labour or confinement in the eighteenth century (Foucault, 1965). It is striking that as lunacy has been reconstructed as illness, its management brought within the professional bounds of medicine, and effective biological treatments developed, views of deviance and 'otherness' remain.

This chapter will examine the way in which those with long-term mental health problems can be voiceless. A limited ability to make their needs known contributes substantially to their ongoing suffering. Analysis of the interaction between mental health difficulties and palliative medicine should identify opportunities to improve the relationship and thereby give this group a greater voice and better care.

Long-term mental health problems

There is a growing awareness of the burden of mental illness within society. One in six adults in the UK is suffering from a mental illness at any one time (Singleton et al., 2001). The last government identified mental health as one of its top three health priorities (Department of Health, 2002) and published national standards for delivery of mental health care (NSF Mental Health, 1999) aiming to 'drive up quality and remove the wide and unacceptable variations in provision'.

Mental illness can be broadly categorized into common mental disorders (CMD) which include depression and anxiety disorders, and severe mental illnesses (SMI)—schizophrenia, bipolar affective disorder, and related psychoses. In addition, addiction and personality difficulties can co-exist with these disorders or present alone. Economically, depression is the greatest mental health problem (Black, 2008). The number of days lost from work and the cost of prescriptions for anti-depressant drugs places a substantial burden on the nation's finances. Anxiety disorders, both discretely and in the context of depression, contribute to individual social disability. Abuse of alcohol and other substances is increasing, at great cost to individuals and society.

The burden of the psychotic disorders, principally schizophrenia, is substantial. The destruction of personality, relationships and social roles is often marked.

Schizophrenia typically develops in the second and third decade and often progresses to a chronic syndrome. The features of the acute syndrome include delusions, where an individual holds usually false beliefs which are unusual in terms of that person's background and are held on inadequate grounds; hallucinations where the individual experiences perceptions in the absence of external stimuli; and disorders of thinking where, for example, the individual will allude to an experience of thoughts which he knows not to be his, or where he perceives his thoughts to be accessible to others without his control. Current anti-psychotic medication is effective at alleviating these symptoms, though relapses can occur at times of stress or if compliance with medication is poor. The chronic syndrome of schizophrenia, which has proved much less amenable to treatment, is characterized by 'negative' symptoms. These include apathy, emotional blunting and social withdrawal in the context of limited or absent insight. Additional depressive features occur in about one third of patients. The lifetime risk of schizophrenia is approximately 1 per cent.

Mental health in palliative care

In recent years, interest in and research into the mental health needs of palliative care patients has developed and depression in particular has been recognized as a common problem requiring detection and treatment (Ly et al., 2002; Rayner et al., 2010). Much research effort has been directed towards identifying those with depression, and studies evaluating interventions have been conducted (Moorey et al., 2008; Strong et al., 2008). Internationally, guidelines are being developed to help clinicians identify, assess and treat depression (EPCRC, 2010). Dementia is now being recognized as a terminal illness in its own right, with specific palliative care needs being identified and addressed (see Chapter 14).

In clinical practice, however, mental health training for palliative care clinicians remains limited, and access to those with expertise in the treatment of mental disorders is reported as difficult (Price et al., 2006). In contrast to the developing interest in common mental disorders and dementia in palliative care, there remains a dearth of available literature addressing the needs of those with severe mental illness in this setting.

General health care for those with long-term mental health problems

Patients with long-term mental health problems are also users of 'physical' health services. Time engaged with palliative medicine is normally preceded by input from primary and, almost certainly, secondary care. Before examining the interface between chronic mental ill health and palliative care, events that occur 'upstream' but which may bias events when the palliative stage is reached, should be understood.

The separation of physical medicine and psychiatric medicine geographically, professionally and, at times, philosophically, produces difficulties for those areas at their interface. In particular this includes patients with unexplained physical symptoms, unloved by physicians and surgeons (Anonymous, 1978), or patients with both medical and psychological pathologies.

Screening for cancer is a good example. Wernecke examined the uptake of breast screening by patients receiving care in a psychiatric hospital (Werneke et al., 2006). Those women with severe mental illness, mainly schizophrenia and bipolar disorder, were significantly less likely to attend breast screening (OR = 0.33, 0.18 to 0.61; p < 0.01).

For symptoms to attract medical attention patients need to 'complain'; a simple step often overlooked. The individual needs to perceive a bodily sensation as concerning, conclude that it requires medical attention and explain this to a doctor. Each of these parts is in turn made up of smaller decisions and actions. A number of the core difficulties of a patient with chronic schizophrenia could prevent one or other of these actions taking place. A suspicious patient, already suffering with unpleasant auditory hallucinations or a belief that another person has control over his thoughts or his bodily functions may not recognize a new physical perception as sinister or requiring medical attention (Talbott and Linn, 1978). The pervasive apathy of the negative syndrome of schizophrenia might prevent that patient seeking medical attention even if he believes it necessary. The difficulties with processing thoughts that interfere with effective communication might prevent the patient accurately describing his symptoms in a way that a doctor would recognize as deserving of further attention.

Physical complaints in patients with known psychiatric disorder can be ascribed to their underlying mental illness, and not given sufficient credence—a phenomenon known as 'diagnostic overshadowing' (Henderson, 2000). Evidence suggests that physicians find psychiatric patients unrewarding (Patel, 1975). Their behavioural problems can make them unwelcome in clinic settings (Karasu et al., 1980). Their difficulties in adhering to management plans can infuriate (McConnell et al., 1992). The sharp division that exists between physical and psychological medicine frequently means that a practitioner in one lacks skills or confidence in examining the other. Liaison psychiatrists have demonstrated that hospital doctors miss psychiatric illness in their patients (Cepoiu et al., 2008), but there is also evidence that psychiatrists are reluctant to physically examine their patients (McIntyre and Romano, 1977).

This inequity is more concerning given that the wider impact of poor mental health on morbidity and mortality (Chafetz et al., 2005). Those with chronic mental illness typically lead less healthy lives. They indulge in more unhealthy activities such as smoking, drinking, and poor diet. They take less exercise, and are more obese. They are more likely to have a range of disorders including cardiovascular disease, raised lipid levels, hypertension, and osteoporosis. In addition, anti-psychotic medication particularly the new generation 'atypical' anti-psychotics can cause weight gain and increase the risk of developing type 2 diabetes (Connolly and Kelly, 2005).

Palliative care for patients with mental health problems

The UK Department of Health End of Life Care strategy (Department of Health, 2008) specifically refers to those with mental health problems at the end of life as a vulnerable group, whose needs may not be identified, resulting in inadequate care.

The Mental Health Foundation review of mental health and palliative care (Ellison, 2008) initially intended to explore general mental health and psychological support for those receiving palliative care. However the authors found a striking gap in the literature concerning the palliative care needs of those with pre-existing mental illness. Of the articles identified which specifically addressed the interface between pre-existing mental health problems and palliative care, one looked at the prevalence of psychiatric disorder in a palliative care unit and found that of 224 admissions over 6 months, 62 per cent met operational criteria for a psychiatric disorder with 1 per cent meeting criteria for schizophrenia or related delusional disorders (Durkin et al., 2003). There were two published case reports describing the care of patients with chronic mental illness at the end of life (Kelly and Shanley, 2000; Candilis and Foti, 1999). Three papers addressed the provision of palliative care for people with serious and persistent mental illness, one by a UK social worker (Davie, 2006) and two from the US, both from a psychiatric nursing perspective (Baker, 2005; McCasland, 2007). These papers emphasized the barriers and challenges to providing good quality palliative care to this population and how each specialty is well placed to make positive changes to current inadequate provision.

Positive Partnerships—Palliative Care for Adults with Severe Mental Health Problems was published jointly by the National Council for Hospice and Specialist Palliative Care Services and Scottish Partnership Agency for Palliative and Cancer Care in 2001 (Addington-Hall, 2000). It addressed the needs of both those with severe and enduring mental illness and those with dementia with life threatening illness requiring palliative care. It aimed to raise awareness among those providing services and facilitate discussion between different agencies as to how these services could be provided. It also provided recommendations and identified research priorities. Recommendations highlighted General Practitioners as key providers and emphasized the importance of partnership working. In palliative care specifically, recommendations were made to provide basic mental health training and training to challenge negative attitudes to those with severe mental illness. It was envisaged that palliative care would mostly take place in the patient's usual place of care.

A systematic review of the literature regarding palliative care for people with severe persistent mental illness (Woods et al., 2008) identified 68 articles in total, mostly from peer reviewed journals, 11 of which contained original data and 57 of which were case reports, commentaries, editorials, or opinion pieces. Of the 11 empirical papers, 3 assessed alcohol use in palliative populations; 4 were concerned with end of life care planning for patients with severe mental illness; 2 used descriptive phenomenology to explore ethico-legal issues in provision of palliative care identified by institutional mental health workers, and palliative care by mental health care workers; one was a descriptive study of shelter-based palliative care for the homeless terminally ill; and one surveyed the attitudes of psychiatrists to palliative care for patients with eating disorders. The review's authors identified four main themes:

- Decision-making and advance care planning
- Access to care
- Provision of care
- Vulnerability.

People with severe mental illness are often not included in end of life discussions due to a presumption of incapacity or fear that such conversations will be destabilizing;

they may also have decisions made on their behalf without consideration of their preferences.

Regarding access to care, people with severe mental illness may experience or respond to physical symptoms differently and delay or not seek appropriate assessment. Their illness may not present in a typical way, or with a history that is difficult to elicit. They may be under-treated as symptoms of medical illness may not be recognized leading to diagnosis at a late stage of illness. Limited or distanced personal relationships may leave patients with a lack of access to support and advocacy.

No coordinated systems are in place for the care of people with severe mental illness at the end of life. Multiple teams and caregivers may be involved but there is little crossover between areas of expertise in end of life care and mental health, resulting in inadequate care in both areas. When palliative care is provided, the presence of a mental illness may present challenges to communication. This could include declining to give a history, consent to examination or tolerating procedures. Social co-morbidities such as homelessness may further complicate provision of care. Palliative care providers may feel under-skilled to provide care for people with severe mental illness and may see this group as outside their areas of expertise or remit. Lack of integrated health care systems may also be detrimental to the care of these patients who have always fared poorly in the transition from predominantly mental health to predominantly physical health care.

Finally people with mental illness have been identified as an especially vulnerable group who find themselves doubly disadvantaged by their combination of physical and mental illness, leading to powerlessness and further diminution of the self at the end of life.

Little literature exists on the bereavement care needs of family and carers of those with mental illness. The death of a loved one who has spent much of their life struggling with mental illness brings particular challenges. As with carers of those with dementia, a kind of social death may have preceded the actual death, but may have happened many years previously. Relatives (most often parents or siblings) may have spent long years dealing with relapses, hospital admissions, social withdrawal, substance use, and other social disadvantages. Bereavement care must be sensitive to individual circumstances and a lack of information and guidance on how to negotiate the particular bereavement issues of this group is a matter of concern.

The literature supports a conclusion that this population is not receiving the care it needs, and furthermore research has largely overlooked them.

New models of service delivery

In an age of austerity with public spending cuts and straightened budgets the most vulnerable members of society will be most affected. This includes those with severe mental illness. There is, however, an ethical and legal duty to provide good quality end of life care to all, regardless of their circumstances and this is enshrined in equalities, capacity and human rights law.

New models of service delivery must provide equality of access to good quality care and reduce stigma experienced by those with severe mental illness. This will require

Table 13.1 Barriers to access to palliative care for people with severe mental illness

Patient factors:

◆ Possible atypical response to/experience of symptoms may lead to delayed/non-help seeking

◆ Atypical illness presentation to health care providers may lead to delayed/non-diagnosis of life limiting illness

◆ History may be difficult to elicit

◆ Possible presence of complex co-morbidities making diagnosis difficult

◆ Limited or distanced personal relationships may result in a lack of advocacy in accessing appropriate services.

Clinician factors:

◆ Attribution of symptoms to mental rather than physical illness (diagnostic overshadowing)

◆ People with severe mental illness may be deemed unsuitable for palliative care services due to a number of factors including behavioural disturbance and challenging social circumstances e.g. homelessness

◆ Lack of exposure to people with severe mental illness leads to reduced confidence in managing this group at the end of life

◆ Negative attitudes toward people with severe mental illness e.g. concerns about violence.

Service-level factors:

◆ Lack of a coordinated system for providing palliative care to people with severe mental illness

◆ Little or no crossover between palliative care and mental health services

◆ Lack of mental health expertise within palliative care services.

education, cross-boundary team working, and a willingness to provide care in a range of settings (Table 13.1).

There is some reason for optimism. In the UK the Department of Health 'e-Learning for Health' programme (eLFH, 2010) has incorporated mental health training sessions into its palliative care programme, allowing those working in the field to develop their skills in recognition, assessment, and management of mental disorders. Training courses for palliative care practitioners which focus on the mental health needs of patients at the end of life have begun. Cross-organizational initiatives such as the Modernisation Initiative End of Life Care Programme (Modernisation Initiative, 2010) are working in partnership with local people, local services and the voluntary sector to improve service delivery to the community. Cross-boundary working is being recognized as a way to improve care when a patient moves from one sector to another within a health service. The following case example illustrates how cross-boundary working can benefit patient care:

Deborah was a 42-year-old lady with a long history of paranoid schizophrenia living in a group home. She had no contact with her family and no friends; however she had a trusting relationship with her key worker and regular contact with her community mental health team. Deborah's symptoms had been stable for over ten years with depot anti-psychotic medication; although her long-standing delusion about parts of her body being controlled by others remained and often led her to report physical symptoms.

When Deborah began to complain of abdominal pain her key worker took her to the GP who attributed her symptoms to her mental illness and reassured her that there was nothing wrong as she had done many times in the past. It was only when her key worker noticed abdominal distension and took her back to the GP that Deborah's symptoms were fully investigated and she was found to have ovarian cancer at an advanced stage.

Deborah's pain was very difficult to manage in the community and she was referred to her local hospice for symptom management. The hospice team were initially reluctant to accept her care because of concern that they would not be able to manage her. However, after discussion with and planned input from the hospice liaison psychiatry team and reassurance from her key worker and community mental health team that they would provide any support needed, she was admitted to the hospice for 2 weeks during which time her pain was brought under control. Her admission was uneventful and her mental state did not deteriorate. After discharge she continued to receive palliative care input from the homecare team until she was re-admitted to the hospice for terminal care and died peacefully.

In the US, the Massachusetts Department of Mental Health have developed a programme in partnership with Palliative Care to integrate end of life planning into mental health care. The programme, 'Do It Your Way' (Foti, 2003), was set up in order to build relationships across mental health and palliative care and is a model of interdisciplinary team working.

Researchers have identified shared qualities and philosophies in mental health and palliative care including a focus on person-centred practice, relationship-based connectedness, and a concern for quality of life as defined by the patient (McGrath and Holewa, 2004); qualities which provide a platform for developing cross-boundary working relationships.

More work is needed however. The Academy of Royal Colleges report *No Health Without Mental Health* (AMRC, 2009) identified a lack of specialist mental health input to palliative care and recommended increasing liaison psychiatry provision, currently a relatively rare resource. The presence of embedded experts within the palliative care setting can improve access and quality of care for those with mental illness, develop links between palliative and mental health services and provide a training resource within services.

Primary care and acute services need to consider referral to palliative care as a realistic option for those with mental illness. Palliative care practitioners need to feel confident to manage patients with mental illness at the end of life. Ongoing training is needed to challenge negative attitudes and reduce anxiety about accepting these patients into palliative care.

Palliative care services can utilize the skills and knowledge of key workers, Community Psychiatric Nurses (CPNs), and others with close professional and carer relationships. In return, mental health services would benefit from the expertise of palliative care practitioners when providing end of life care to their patients. Building on ideas of cross-boundary working, reciprocity of skills, and shared care will be crucial to providing good quality end of life care either in both in-patient and community settings.

Recognition of the individual needs of carers and family of a person with chronic mental illness provides particular challenges for bereavement care. It is of concern that so little research has been done in this area. The field of palliative care for people with severe mental illness is 'wide open' in terms of research potential (Woods et al., 2008) and there is much opportunity for further work on the palliative care needs of this vulnerable and overlooked group.

Resources

- ◆ MIND. Information and advice.
  www.mind.org.uk/help/information_and_advice
- ◆ Mental Health Foundation.
  www.mentalhealth.org.uk/information/
- ◆ Royal College of Psychiatrists. Mental health information for all.
  www.rcpsych.ac.uk/mentalhealthinfo.aspx

References

Academy of Medical Royal Colleges. (2009). *No Health Without Mental Health*. London: Royal College of Psychiatristsl.

Addington-Hall, J. (2000). *Positive Partnerships: Palliative Care for Adults with Severe Mental Health Problems*. London: National Council for Hospice and Specialist Palliative Care Services and Scottish Partnership Agency for Palliative and Cancer Care, Occasional Paper 17.

Anonymous. (1978). Taking care of the hateful patient. *N Engl J Med*, **299**: 366–7.

Baker, A. (2005). Palliative and end-of-life care in the serious and persistently mentally ill population. *Journal of the American Psychiatric Nurses Association*, **11**: 298.

Black, C. (2008). *Working for a Healthier Tomorrow*. London: The Stationery Office.

Candilis, P. and Foti, M. E. (1999). Case presentation: End-of-life care and mental illness: The case of Ms. W. *Journal of Pain and Symptom Management*, **18**: 447–8.

Cepoiu, M., McCusker, J., Cole, M. G., Sewitch, M., Belzile, E., and Ciampi, A. (2008). Recognition of depression by non-psychiatric physicians—A systematic literature review and meta-analysis. *J Gen Intern Med*, **23**: 25–36.

Chafetz, L., White, M., Collins-Bride, G., and Nickens, J. (2005). The poor general health of the severely mentally ill: Impact of schizophrenic diagnosis. *Community Mental Health J*, **41**: 169–84.

Connolly, M. and Kelly, C. (2005). Lifestyle and physical health in schizophrenia. *Advances in Psychiatric Treatment*, **11**: 125–32.

Davie, E. (2006). A social work perspective on palliative care for people with mental health problems. *European Journal of Palliative Care*, **13**: 26–8.

Department of Health. (2002). *Saving Lives: Our Healthier Nation*. London: Department of Health.

Department of Health. (2008). *End of life Care Strategy*. London: Department of Health.

Durkin, I., Kearney, M., and O'Siorain, L. (2003). Psychiatric disorder in a palliative care unit. *Palliat Med*, **17**: 212–18.

e-Learning for Healthcare, available at: www.e-lfh.org.uk.

Ellison, N. (2008). *Mental Health and Palliative Care Literature Review*. London: The Mental Health Foundation.

European Palliative Care Research Collaborative. (2010). *Guidelines for Assessment and Treatment of Depression in Palliative Care*. Available at: www.epcrc.org.

Foti, M. (2003). Do it your way: A demonstration on end-of-life care for persons with serious mental illness. *Journal of Palliative Medicine*, **6**: 661–9.

Foucault, M. (1965). *Madness and Civilisation, A History of Insanity in the Age of Reason*. New York: Random House.

Henderson, M. (2000). A difficult psychiatric patient. *Postgrad Med J*, **76**: 590–1.

Karasu, T., Waltzman, S., Lindenmayer, J., and Buckley, P. (1980). The medical care of patients with psychiatric illness. *Hosp Community Psychiatry*, **31**: 463–72.

Kelly, B. and Shanley, D. (2000). Terminal illness and schizophrenia *J Palliat Care*, **16**: 55–57.

Ly, K., Chidgey, J., Addington-Hall, J., and Hotopf, M. (2002). Depression in palliative care: A systematic review, Part 2, Treatment. *Palliat Med*, **16**: 279–84.

McCasland, L. (2007). Providing hospice and palliative care to the seriously and persistently mentally ill. *Journal of Hospice & Palliative Nursing*, **9**: 305–13.

McConnell, S. D., Inderbitzin, L. B., and Pollard, W. E. (1992). Primary health care in the CMHC: A role for the nurse practitioner. *Hosp Community Psychiatry*, **43**: 724–7.

McGrath, P. and Holewa, H. (2004). Mental health and palliative care: Exploring the ideological interface. *Int J Psychosoc Rehabil*, **9**(1): 107–19.

McIntyre, J. and Romano, J. (1977). Is there a stethoscope in the house (and is it used)? *Arch Gen Psychiatry*, **34**: 1147–51.

Modernisation Initiative End of life Care Project. Located at Guys and St Thomas' Charity, London.

Moorey, S., Cort, E., Kapari, M., Monroe, B., Hansford, P., Mannix, K., et al. (2008). A cluster randomized controlled trial of cognitive behaviour therapy for common mental disorders in patients with advanced cancer. *Psychol Med*, **39**(5): 713–23.

National Service Frameworks, Mental Health: Modern Standards and Service Models. (1999). London, Department of Health.

Patel, A. (1975). Attitudes towards self-poisoning *Br Ned J*, **2**: L426–9.

Price, A., Hotopf, M., Higginson, I., Monroe, B., and Henderson, M. (2006). Psychological services in hospices in the UK and Republic of Ireland. *J R Soc Med*, **99**: 637–9.

Rayner, L., Lee, W., Price, A., Evans, A., Koravangattu, V., Higginson, I. J., et al. (2010). The clinical epidemiology of depression in palliative care and the predicative value of somatic symptoms; cross survey and four week follow up. *Palliative Medicine* (in press).

Singleton, N., Bumpstead, R., O'Brien, M., Lee, A., and Meltzer, H. (2001). Psychiatric morbidity among people living in private households, 2000. London: The Stationery Office.

Strong, V., Waters, R., Hibberd, C., Murray, G., Wall, L., Walker, J., et al. (2008). Management of depression for people with cancer (SMaRT oncology 1): A randomised trial. *Lancet*, **372**: 40–8.

Talbott, J., and Linn, L. (1978). Reactions of schizophrenics to life-threatening disease. *Psychiat Q*, **50**: 218–27.

Werneke, U., Horn, O., Maryon-Davis, A., Wessely, S., Donnan, S., and McPherson, K. (2006). Uptake of screening for breast cancer in patients with mental health problems. *JECH*, **60**: 600–5.

Woods, A., Willison, K., Kington, C., and Gavin, A. (2008). Palliative care for people with severe persistent mental illness: A review of the literature. *Canadian Journal of Psychiatry*, **53**: 725–36.

Chapter 14

People with dementia

Murna Downs

Context

Dementia is a syndrome, or collection of symptoms, characterized by progressive cognitive and functional impairment caused by progressive brain diseases. As such, it is more accurate to think of the *dementias* as a group of progressive brain diseases, the most common of which are Alzheimer's disease and vascular dementia, than *dementia* as a single disease entity.

Dementia is most common in those over 65 with approximately 5% of those over 65 and 20% of those over 80 having some kind of dementia. As the biggest risk factor for developing dementia is old age, growth in the number of people with dementia is associated with growth in those over 65, and in particular those over 80 (Ferri et al., 2005; WHO, 2009). With declining fertility and rising longevity, those over 80 are now the fastest growing age group in society (WHO, 2009).

It is widely recognized that the number of people with dementia will grow throughout the world (Ferri et al., 2005). As of 2010 there were nearly 36 million people living with dementia and this number is expected to double every 20 years to 66 million by 2030 and to more than 115 million by 2050 (Alzheimer's Disease International, 2009). While the increase in the number of people with dementia will be greatest in developing countries (Ferri et al., 2005), growth in numbers will also effect European countries (WHO, 2009).

A significant minority of people also develop dementia below the age of 65, called 'early onset dementia', and this requires attention in its own right. In addition, prevalence of dementia is higher in people with learning disabilities than in the general population, particularly those with Down's syndrome.

Dementia is a major cause of disability and dependence (Moise et al., 2004), with significant human and economic costs. Most people with dementia live at home with their families who, in turn, provide most of the day-to-day care and support. Of the 700,000 people with dementia in the UK, almost two-thirds live in their own homes, usually with their family carers. Consequently, dementia affects both the person with dementia and their family members. The health-related consequences of poorly supported family care have been extensively documented throughout the world (Alzheimer's Disease International, 2009). In England the need to provide proactive support to family carers is recognized within the National Dementia Strategy (Department of Health, 2009a) which is intended to articulate closely with the National Carers' Strategy (Department of Health, 2008).

The costs of formal and informal care for people with dementia and their families are enormous and are set to grow in line with the number of people with dementia (Wimo et al., 2007). The total estimated world-wide costs of dementia are $604 billion in 2010 (Alzheimer's Disease International, 2010). As such, dementia has been described as one of the greatest public health problems of our time (Wimo et al., 2007). Costs to the UK economy are estimated at approximately £23 billion a year (Alzheimer's Research Trust, 2010).

Dementia is not only associated with significant financial costs, but also with significant personal and social costs. The stigma, discrimination, and social exclusion experienced by people with dementia and their families have been documented (Graham et al., 2003). Indeed it has been argued that the social consequences constitute a malignancy in their own right (Kitwood, 1997). As a consequence many of the national plans for dementia have identified combating stigma as a priority (International Journal of Geriatric Psychiatry: *The Challenges of Dementia: An International Perspective*, 2010).

Needs of people with dementia at end of life

People with advanced dementia can live for several years dependent on others for all aspects of their care—physical, emotional, psychological, social, and spiritual.

Promoting physical health and well-being

A key aspect to physical comfort and well-being is the assessment and treatment of pain. It has been well documented that people with dementia are less likely to have their pain treated than are people without dementia who have similar physical conditions, including hip fracture (Morrison and Siu, 2000). Sampson and colleagues, in a retrospective case review, demonstrated that people with dementia who died in hospital were less likely than cognitively intact counterparts to receive palliative medications or be referred to palliative care teams prior to death (Sampson et al., 2006).

People with advanced dementia require opportunities for movement and thoughtful positioning. Adequate attention to the need for movement can help prevent skin breakdown and pressure sores. Oral care is required to prevent mouth ulcers and thrush which can be painful. Despite a lack of evidence to support their use (Sampson et al., 2009), feeding tubes are used with people with advanced dementia.

Holmes, Sachs et al. (2008), using a Delphi consensus method, demonstrated a worrying frequency of polypharmacy and inappropriate prescribing for people with advanced dementia. They argue for the need for consensus criteria to ensure the appropriate prescription of medication to this client group, in particular weighing the risks against potential benefits.

Personal care includes help with eating, drinking, positioning, dressing, bathing, and toileting. As the person with dementia becomes less and less able to care for him or herself s/he will require help with every aspect of care. Such assistance provides the care staff and person opportunities for engagement. We know that a person who requires help in this way retains awareness of their social place and value. It is essential that care is provided such that it affirms personhood rather than in a mechanistic, depersonalized way.

Promoting emotional, social, and spiritual well-being

It is in the area of care of people with advanced dementia that the thorny issues of what it means to be human which so engaged Kitwood (1997) are most evident. It is now recognized that people with advanced dementia continue to have human needs. Both philosophical arguments and a growing body of empirical evidence support this position of retained personhood in advanced dementia.

Norberg and colleagues (1986) led the field in demonstrating empirically the extent to which awareness and capacity for communication are retained in people with severe dementia. Their work amply demonstrates that communication difficulties at the end of life have as much to do with our lack of understanding of alternative forms of expression as with the person's difficulty with verbal expression.

People with limited or no language will often express themselves through their behaviour (Cohen-Mansfield, 2008). The concept of 'need-driven compromised behaviour' is increasingly being applied to understanding behavioural aspects of dementia. In this way the notion of 'challenging behaviour' as being a 'symptom' of dementia is being replaced with a concern with identifying what need the behaviour is seeking to meet (Algase et al., 1996).

Clare and colleagues (2008) have demonstrated significant levels of awareness in people with dementia living in care homes. Kontos (2005), from a sociology of the body perspective, has demonstrated 'embodied selfhood' in people with advanced dementia. Increasingly it is recognized that knowledge of a person's life story, life long needs and preferences is essential to quality end of life care. Creative arts are being used to facilitate self expression and affirm personhood in people with advanced dementia.

The religious and spiritual needs of people with dementia are often neglected. For example, in a retrospective case review of people who died with and without dementia in an acute ward, people with dementia were less likely than people without to have mention of their religious faith in their case notes. Only three of these patients had had any assessment of their spiritual needs (Sampson et al., 2006).

Needs of families at end of life

It is now widely recognized that family should have the opportunity to take their rightful place as partners in care of their relative, as well as having their own needs for support and information met. Yet the literature is littered with the neglect of family perspectives and experience and expertise which the Nolan et al. (2004) relationship-centred care strives to address.

Care for people with advanced dementia often places the family in the role of decision-maker and much can be done to minimize the stress associated with this role. Family conflict is not unusual at this time. Preventing and addressing family conflict can be achieved with facilitated family meetings (see for example Zarit and Zarit, 2007). There is also a need to address communication between families and professionals regarding end of life care (Levenson, 2004). Partnership working is poorly developed leading to 'lose lose' rather than 'win win' scenarios.

Needs of staff caring at end of life

There is increasing evidence in the literature that care staff who provide most of the day to day care to people with advanced dementia are often economic migrants. This creates its own challenges as care workers bring their own nuanced cultural understandings, language, and religion to bear on the end of life care which may be at odds with the mores and norms of the host country.

It is now recognized that care home staff are poorly prepared for their role in supporting people with dementia (All Party Parliamentary Group, 2009). This is even more pronounced for those who work with the person with advanced dementia. They require specialist training and education, including in end of life and palliative care, along with emotional support and supervision. Even though national policy favours a person-centred approach, it is clear that the emotional side of care work is often not considered a legitimate part of the job. This is particularly necessary at the time of a resident's death and adopting a 'family' approach is recommended (Moss et al., 2003).

Issues at end of life care

There are several issues concerning end of life care for people with dementia and their families including:

- ◆ Recognition of advanced dementia as a terminal illness
- ◆ Reconsidering the need for prognostication of the terminal phase
- ◆ Establishing evidence-based care standards and outcomes
- ◆ Decision-making and advance planning.

Recognition of advanced dementia as a terminal illness

One of the issues in end of life care for people with dementia is that advanced dementia is not universally seen as a terminal illness (Mitchell et al., 2009). Perhaps one of the implications of dementia being classed as a mental health (neuro-psychiatric) problem of old age is that its neurological toll on the body and its functions is less well understood and supported (Downs et al., 2006; Mitchell et al., 2009).

Reconsider the need for prognostication of the terminal phase

Predicting or identifying the terminal phase in advanced dementia is notoriously difficult, wrong about one-third of the time (Mitchell et al., 2010). Yet such prognostication is often required for the introduction of palliative and hospice services. As a result Mitchell and colleagues plead that comfort and palliative care should be accessible to all people with advanced dementia. Such support would ensure the provision of psychological, social and spiritual support to people with dementia and their families. It would ensure that people who do eventually die with dementia are prevented the unnecessary suffering associated with undetected and untreated pain, shortness of breath and futile hospitalizations (Mitchell et al., 2010).

Establish evidence-based care standards and compliance monitoring

Despite growing numbers of people dying with and from dementia, we have a relatively underdeveloped evidence base of best practice in this area. Most of our research has identified shortcomings in current approaches. What the field now needs is evidence-based guidance on best practice and mechanisms for ensuring its implementation.

Decision-making and advance planning

The Department of Health's (2009a) *National Dementia Strategy* places significant emphasis on improving the end of life care for people with dementia. Its main suggestion for achieving this is to involve people with dementia and their carers in planning end of life care, recognizing the principles outlined in the Department of Health's (2009b) *End of Life Care Strategy*. As such, it is really focussed on terminal care. Advance care planning has a role to play in ensuring quality terminal care, but it by no means guarantees it. The recent report from the Nuffield Council on Bioethics (2009) describes the limitations of advance care planning. In addition, Dekkers (2004) argues for us to think about bodily autonomy when considering people's preferences for end of life care.

Examples of best practice

Care at home

See detailed description of care at home until the end of life by old age psychiatrist Adrian Treolar and his team (2009).

See the story of Barbara Pointon caring for her husband Malcolm at home until he died: http://alzheimers.org.uk/site/scripts/news_article.php?newsID=99.

Care in care homes

Examples of innovations in care homes can be found on the End of Life Care programme website:www.endoflifecareforadults.nhs.uk/case-studies/improving-eolc-dementia-north-west.And see also the National End of Life Care Intelligence Network Report on Dementia (9 Nov. 2010).

Resources

- ◆ Hughes, J. C. (ed.) (2005). *Palliative care in Severe Dementia*. London: Quay Books.
- ◆ Volicer, L. (2005). *End of Life Care for People with Dementia in Residential Care Settings*. US Alzheimer's Association. www.alz.org/national/documents/endoflifelitreview.pdf.
- ◆ The (Australian) National Palliative Care Programme. (2006). *Guidelines for a Palliative Approach in Residential Aged Care*. www.nhmrc.gov.au/_files_nhmrc/file/publications/synopses/pc29.pdf.
- ◆ Pace, V., Treolar, A., and Scott, S. (In press). *Dementia: From Advanced Disease to Bereavement*. Oxford Specialist Handbook in End of Life Care. Oxford: Oxford University Press.

References

Algase, D. L., Beck, C., Kolanowski, A., Whall, A., Berent, S., Richards, K., et al. (1996). Need-driven dementia-compromised behavior: An alternative view of disruptive behavior. *American Journal of Alzheimer's Disease and Other Dementias,* **11**: 10–19.

All Party Parliamentary Group on Dementia. (2009). *Prepared to Care: Challenging the Dementia Skills Gap.* London: All Party Parliamentary Group on Dementia [web publication].

Alzheimer's Disease International. (2009). *World Alzheimer report.* London: Alzheimer's Disease International.

Alzheimer's Disease International. (2010). *World Alzheimer Report: The Global Economic Impact of Dementia.* London: Alzheimer's Disease International.

Alzheimer's Research Trust. (2010). *Dementia 2010.* www.dementia2010.org.

Clare, L., Rowlands, J., Bruce, E., Surr, C., and Downs, M. (2008). 'I don't do like I used to do': A grounded theory approach to conceptualizing awareness in people with moderate to severe dementia living in long-term care. *Social Science and Medicine,* **66**(11): 2366–77.

Cohen-Mansfield, J. (2008). Understanding the language of behaviour. In M. Downs and B. Bowers (eds), *Excellence in Dementia Care: Research into Practice.* Maidenhead, UK: Open University Press, 187–211.

Dekkers, W. J. M. (2004). Autonomy and the lived body in cases of severe dementia. In R. B. Purtilo and H. A. M. J. Ten Have (eds), *Ethical Foundations of Palliative Care for Alzheimer Disease.* London: Johns Hopkins University Press.

Department of Health. (2008). *Carers at the Heart of 21st-century Families and Communities. 'A Caring System on Your Side. A Life of Your Own.'* London: The Stationery Office.

Department of Health. (2009a). *Living Well with Dementia: A National Dementia Strategy.* London: The Stationery Office.

Department of Health. (2009b). *End of life care strategy.* London: The Stationery Office.

Downs, M., Small, N., and Froggatt, K. (2006). Explanatory models of dementia: Links to end-of-life care. *International Journal of Palliative Nursing,* **12**(5): 209–13.

Ferri, C. P., Prince, M., Brayne, C., Brodaty, H., Fratiglioni, L., Ganguli, M., et al., (2005). Global prevalence of dementia: A Delphi consensus study. *The Lancet,* **366**(9503): 2112–17.

Graham, N., Lindesay, J., Katona, C., Bertolote, J. M., Camus, V., Copeland, J. et al. (2003). Reducing stigma and discrimination against older people with mental disorders: A technical consensus statement. *International Journal of Geriatric Psychiatry,* **18**(8): 670–8.

Holmes, H. M., Sachs, G., Shega, J. W., Hougham, G. W., Hayley, D. C., and Dale, W. (2008). Integrating palliative medicine into the care of persons with advanced dementia: Identifying appropriate medication use. *Journal of the American Geriatrics Society,* **56**(7): 1306–11.

International Journal of Geriatric Psychiatry. (Sept. 2010). *The Challenges of Dementia: An International Perspective.*

Kitwood, T. (1997). *Dementia Reconsidered: The Person Comes First.* Buckingham, UK: Open University Press.

Kontos, P. (2005). Embodied selfhood in Alzheimer's disease: Rethinking person-centred care. *Dementia,* **4**(4): 553–70.

Levenson, R. (2004). Lessons from the end of life. *British Medical Journal,* **329**(7476): 1244.

Mitchell, S., Miller, S., Teno, J. M., Kiely, D. K., Davis, R. B., Shaffer, M. L. (2010). Prediction of 6-month survival of nursing home residents with advanced dementia using ADEPT vs hospice eligibility guidelines. *Journal of the American Medical Association,* **304**(17): 1929–35.

Mitchell, S. L., Teno, J. M., Kiely, D. K., Shaffer, M. L., Jones, R. N., Prigerson, H. G., et al. (2009). The clinical course of advanced dementia. *N Engl J Med*, **361**(16): 1529–38.

Moise, P., Schwarzinger, M., Um, M.-Y., et al. (2004). *Dementia Care in 9 OECD Countries. A Comparative Analysis.* Paris: OECD; 2004. OECD Health Working Papers No. 13.

Morrison, R. S. and Siu, A. L. (2000). A comparison of pain and its treatment in advanced dementia and cognitively intact patients with hip fracture. *Journal of Pain and Symptom Management*, **19**(4): 240–8.

Moss, M. S., Moss, S. Z. Rubinstein, R. L., and Black, H. K. (2003). The metaphor of 'family' in staff communication about dying and death. *Journal of Gerontology, Psychological Science Social Science*, **58**(5): S290–6.

Nolan, M. R., Davies, S., Brown, J., Keady, J., and Nolan, J. (2004). Beyond 'person-centred' care: A new vision for gerontological nursing. *International Journal of Older People Nursing*, **13**(3a): 45–53.

Norberg, A., Melin, E., and Asplund, K. (1986). Reactions to music, touch and object presentation in the final stage of dementia: An exploratory study. *International Journal of Nursing Studies*, **23**(4): 315–23.

Nuffield Council on Bioethics. (2009). *Dementia: Ethical Issues.* London: Nuffield Council on Bioethics.

Sampson, E. L., Candy, B., and Jones, L. (2009). *Enteral Tube Feeding for Older People with Advanced Dementia.* Cochrane Database Systematic Review, CD007209.

Sampson, E. L., Gould, V., Lee, D., and Blanchard, M. (2006). Differences in care received by patients with and without dementia who died during acute hospital admission: A retrospective case note study. *Age and Ageing*, **8** (2): 187–9.

Treolar, A., Crugel, M., and Adamis, D. (2009). Palliative and end of life care of dementia at home is feasible and rewarding: Results from the Hope for Home study. *Dementia*, **8**(3): 335–47.

Wimo, A., Winblad, B., and Jönsson, L. (2007). An estimate of the total worldwide societal costs of dementia in 2005. *Alzheimer's and Dementia*, **3**: 81–91.

World Health Organization. (2009). *Mental Health in the EU Context: Dementia and Alzheimers.* New York: WHO.

Zarit, S. H. and Zarit, J. M. (2007). *Mental Disorders in Older Adults*, 2nd edn. New York: Guilford.

Chapter 15

Homeless people

Louise Jones

Context

When we think of a homeless person, what image comes to mind? A shapeless figure huddled in a doorway surrounded by newspaper and cardboard boxes? An ill-kempt character in poorly-fitting clothes carrying their worldly goods in a few plastic bags? A straggle of elderly men on park benches with beer cans for company? Yet homeless people are not so different from others except in the particular mixture of life events and characteristics that have led them sometimes to choose, more often to drift into, this way of life.

Being homeless is often part of social exclusion and a symptom of more fundamental problems. Many homeless people have survived difficult backgrounds, served in the armed forces or spent time in prison; maintaining close ties may be a challenge, and relationship failure is common. Such personal and family circumstances may lead people to sleep rough. Over time, these factors are often compounded by a complex blend of mental and physical illness, and abuse of drugs including alcohol. However, homeless people are just as worthy of respect and opportunities for success as any other group in society.

Numbers

It is difficult to be sure of the total number of people that are homeless as the population is often transient. People sleeping rough may bed down at different times, move about, be hidden away in derelict buildings or travel on all-night buses. The main sources of published data in the UK are street counts of those sleeping rough, local authority figures on the numbers applying to them as homeless, or statistics from specialized agencies on the numbers of clients they serve.

In the 1990s, the voluntary sector and the UK government agreed to use regular street counts in a consistent though incomplete way (www.communities.gov.uk/housing/homelessness/roughsleeping/). Thus, it is estimated that in England in 2009 an average of 464 people were sleeping rough on any given night, of whom 265 (57%) were in London. Additional figures from CHAIN (2009), a London-based recording system, suggest that throughout 2009 a total of 3,472 people were seen rough sleeping in the capital of whom 87% were male, 61% were aged 26–45 years, 49% were white British, 62% of UK nationality, 14% were nationals of recent EU accession, and as many as 31% were from black and ethnic minority groups. Across England, 183 day centres serve an estimated 10,000 people per day, and there are 263 direct access hostels and second stage accommodation projects attempting to meet the needs of the homeless (Homeless Link, 2009).

Provision

There are a number of organizations in the UK providing care and support to homeless people. Well-known examples include: the Salvation Army (www.salvationarmy. org.uk/); Centrepoint, which focuses on young people (www.centrepoint.org.uk/); the Simon Community where workers live closely with their clients (www.simoncommunity.org.uk/); Crisis (www.crisis.org.uk/); Thamesreach (www.thamesreach.org. uk/); and St Mungo's (www.mungos.org/). All have similar aims, but slightly different strategies.

♦ Crisis supports a number of schemes in UK cities (e.g. City Skylight Centres) and aims to improve education, employment, housing and well-being for the single homeless.

♦ Thamesreach supports 3,500 homeless people per year, providing a range of services and using key workers to coordinate health and social care. Approximately 17% of its workforce were formerly homeless. Originating in London, it now offers a national consultancy service.

♦ St Mungo's provides accommodation for up to 1,500 people every night in emergency shelters, hostels, supported housing, and outreach services, mainly in London and the south of England. A recovery approach is used, with outreach and inreach support.

Health needs

It is known that in the UK and USA homeless people are frequent users of Accident and Emergency services, particularly in the days and weeks before death when their health has become critical (O'Connell, 2005; DH, 2010).

Conducting meaningful research to explore their multiple and complex needs is challenging. Capacity to give informed consent may fluctuate due to variations in mental health status and poly-substance abuse. Cross-sectional studies may be possible, but longitudinal follow-up is hampered by itinerant lifestyles and difficulties in achieving future meetings, easily forgotten by clients.

The Salvation Army completed a cross-sectional study involving 438 homeless people in 19 residential or day centres across the UK in 2006–8 (Bonner, www.salvationarmy. org.uk/). This revealed that for most of their lives many had had few friends and limited contact with family members. More than half spent most of their time alone, however only 25% found this unacceptable. Evidence is poorly recorded, but this isolation may be linked to negative or abusive relationships in early life. In exploring mental health, 42% reported post traumatic stress disorder, 22% psychosis, and 17% had significant personality disorder. Of those with post traumatic stress disorder, 30% attributed this to an experience of death or grief, 20% an abusive or neglectful experience in childhood, and 11% to family breakdown. Those with psychosis and personality disorder were more likely to have a history of involvement in violent and non-violent crime.

A survey of clients accessing services provided by St Mungo's in 2009 found that more than two-thirds had issues with substance abuse (alcohol and/or drugs) including mental health problems such as depression and self harm. In addition, 66% had a physical health condition or required regular medication, 52% had educational needs (learning disabilities and literacy and numeracy problems), 48% were ex-offenders and 11% had a history of being in care during their childhood. Making sense of these figures, it becomes apparent that more than two-thirds of clients had multiple needs, often termed 'trimorbidity', most commonly combinations of substance abuse, mental illness, and a variety of physical health problems (O'Connell, 2005; DH, 2010). Given these complex challenges, homeless people are at least three times more likely than the general population to die at any time. We know that the average age of people who die whilst in hostels or registered with homeless services is 40–4 years, but these figures discount those who later become settled in a home and therefore do not indicate life expectancy. The main causes of death are reported as cardiac disease, liver failure, cancer and respiratory illness such as pneumonia. Research by Crisis has shown that the risk of suicide is 35 times that of the general population.

Barriers to end of life care

Despite the acknowledgement of inequalities for homeless people (DH, 2008), significant barriers to improvement remain. For example, in primary care it may not be possible without a permanent address to access services or register with a doctor, and lack of an informal caregiver may impede delivery of care (Mahoney et al., 2008). Hostels that encourage maximum independent living may be listed as private addresses and professionals may not be aware of the high risk status of some of their patients. These issues may be compounded by discrimination from health care professionals on grounds of racial background, HIV or hepatitis C status, and substance abuse (Tarzian, Neal, and O'Neil, 2005). Homeless people may be distrusting of professionals, fearful that abstinence from drugs and alcohol will be a condition of accessing treatment, and drug users may fear that requests for pain relief will be viewed as drug-seeking behaviour (Moller, 2005; Podymow, Turnbull, and Coyle 2006; Kushel and Miakowski, 2006).

End of life care preferences

Our understanding of the experiences of homeless people dying on the streets, in shelters or in hospital remains poor. A systematic review of the limited literature found that many homeless people are unable to access palliative care until very late in their illness, their choices for care are reduced and most die within secondary care (Ahmed et al., 2004). A qualitative study in which 53 homeless people in Minnesota USA discussed their views on end of life care found that many expressed a wish to have someone with them, although this might be a stranger since family members may not be available (Song et al., 2007).

Research from north America on barriers to accessing end of life care for homeless people, the preferences they may have and what facilities currently exist that are specific to their needs, has shown that the life experiences of homeless people, such as repeated bereavements, are likely to influence their attitudes to death and dying (Tarzian, Neal, and O'Neil, 2005). When asked about their concerns, many expressed fear of dying anonymously or undiscovered as well as ambivalence about contacting family members even when they might be aware that their health is deteriorating.

However, if invited to plan for end of life care, many viewed this as a favourable option, providing opportunities for expressing their own wishes, something which may not often have been possible during their lives (Song et al., 2007, 2008).

End of life care provision

Palliative care provision must be sufficiently flexible to accommodate complex needs. In UK, the relative independence of many hospices allows a person-centred approach that can be tailored for those who are homeless. One group of homeless people suggested a dedicated half-way house shelter, staffed 24 hours a day, to provide a safe convalescent environment on leaving hospital (Song et al., 2007). This idea has been successfully piloted in Ottawa, Canada, where homeless clients found the service helpful and much preferable to hospital (Podymow, Turnbull, and Coyle, 2006). Such a facility might be more economically viable if widely used by residents recovering from acute or chronic episodes of illness or injury, reducing expensive hospital admissions (Cagle, 2009).

Example of good practice

St Mungo's and the UK's largest voluntary end of life care provider, Marie Curie Cancer Care (www.mariecurie.org.uk/), have explored ways to improve end of life care for homeless people. Backed by short-term government funding, a palliative care coordinator has worked directly with residents known to be dying from any diagnosis. The role involves strengthening local links with palliative care services. In addition, extra support is offered to hostel staff, helping them to recognize signs of approaching death and improving their confidence in dealing with personal issues for residents, their families, and for themselves.

On average, about 30 people each year die while resident in St Mungo's accommodation. Reported causes of death include cardiac and respiratory diseases (such as pneumonia), and some residents commit suicide. However, the largest factor contributing to death is liver disease, usually related to a history of chronic alcohol abuse. Most deaths are perceived by hostel staff as occurring suddenly, even if they were not entirely unexpected.

Looking deeper

A deeper understanding is needed of how homeless people in the UK perceive their deteriorating condition. As a start, researchers from the Marie Curie unit at University College London have conducted a detailed review of the case notes held by St Mungo's for deaths related to liver disease resulting from alcohol abuse that occurred in 2009/10. Of the 21 cases reviewed so far, most were male, the average age was 57 years and 13 were ex-offenders; all had a history of alcohol abuse and 13 also had a history of drug use. The most common mental health problems were depression and poor memory. In the

6 months before death, 17 had been admitted to hospital of whom five had been admitted at least 3 times; the average length of stay during the final admission was 10 days. Two-thirds of deaths occurred in hospital. The most commonly reported symptoms were poor memory and appetite, feeling unwell, pain, withdrawal fits, abdominal distension, jaundice, nausea and vomiting, and bleeding from the mouth and rectum.

Some marked changes in behaviour were observed. Almost half increased their alcohol consumption in the weeks before death; approximately one-third showed a mixed picture of low mood, poor hygiene, taking to their beds, or becoming anxious to re-connect with family or friends. Health care records were not accessed in this review but there was little evidence of residents accessing primary or palliative care services, or exploring preferences for care or advance care planning, although some had been warned by health professionals that they would die if they did not stop drinking. Although residents may have been internally conscious that they were nearing the end of their lives, this was not often communicated to those around them and opportunities to access health care support were frequently missed. Enlightened by these findings it may be possible to plan pragmatic studies to collect data directly from homeless people on their hopes and fears as death approaches.

Pathway picture

The complex pattern of typical events in the last six months of life of homeless people with liver failure is illustrated in the flow diagram in Figure 15.1 (Davis et al., 2011).

Living in the real world

Improved end of life care for the homeless population requires a flexible approach that takes into account the particular challenges faced and presented by this client group. It is unrealistic to imagine that many individuals will connect regularly with primary or palliative care providers for assessment or symptom control. When acutely ill, or in need of additional care, many will seek treatment from the emergency services.

However, it may be possible for staff in hostels to recognize key changes either in behaviour or symptom burden that provide clues that death is near. Such awareness may enable hostel staff to encourage residents to begin to discuss what might be happening to them, or to explore and facilitate opportunities for reconciliation with family or friends. This may increase the chance of a dignified death and ease the path of both the dying and the bereaved. An approach of competent and compassionate care is supported by a 'route to success' document produced by the National End of Life Care programme (Route to Success Series. www.endofolifecareforadults.nhs.uk).

Improving our understanding

Taking account of user views in the development of interventions in health care enhances effectiveness (Candy, 2010). More research to hear how homeless people themselves suggest that their needs could be met would challenge unrealistic assumptions about

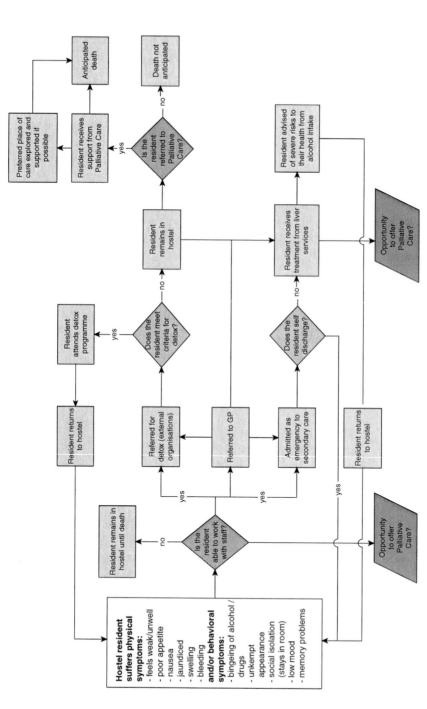

Fig. 15.1 Pathway for homeless people with liver failure. This flow diagram illustrates what commonly occurs in the last few weeks of life for homeless people with liver disease as frequently observed by professionals working in the field. It describes key points at which decisions on future care might be considered, including opportunities for palliative care interventions. (Reproduced from Davis et al. (2011), with permission.)

what is best for them, and inform the planning and delivery of pragmatic interventions that make appropriate use of scarce resources.

Supporting those who work with homeless people

In addition to building on the work of the St Mungo's/Marie Curie approach, there are other ways in which health and social care staff can liaise for the benefit of homeless people. One example of good practice is the model used by Thamesreach where a key worker is dedicated to the integrated care of an individual homeless person. This approach attempts to tackle distrust of health professionals and poor attendance at clinic or primary care appointments to access care.

Some projects provide structured input from medical professionals through regular in-house surgeries in their hostels. This may offer the opportunity for homeless people, hostel or clinical staff to highlight issues of concern and open up possibilities of realistic approaches to future care. Many projects also provide regular supervision sessions with their staff, aiming to minimize any distress which may result from difficult situations around the end of life for homeless people and their families.

Resources

◆ Route to Success Series found at www.endoflifecareforaults.nhs.uk.
◆ Contact Peter.Kennedy@mungos.org for advice on training to provide support at the end of life.
◆ Davis, S., Greenish, W., Kennedy, P., Jones, L. (2011). Improving the management of the end of life in homeless people with advanced liver disease. Report, Marie Curie Cancer Care and St Mungo's. www.mariecurie.org.uk http://www.mungos.org/.

Acknowledgements

I would like to thank Sarah Davis and Wendy Greenish for their help in compiling data for this chapter.

References

Ahmed, N., Bestall, J., Ahmedzai, S., Payne, S., Clark, D., and Noble, B. (2004). Systematic review of the problems and issues accessing specialist palliative care by patients, carers and health and social care professionals. *Palliative Medicine,* **18**: 525–42.

Bonner, A. and Luscombe, C. (2010). The Seeds of Exclusion. ISBN 978–0-85412–788-7, www.salvationarmy.org.uk/.

Cagle, J., (2009). Weathering the storm: Palliative care and elderly homeless persons. *Journal of Housing for the Elderly,* **23**(1): 29–46.

Candy, B. (2010). Systematic reviews of complex interventions: A new approach using qualitative synthesis to analyse trial evidence. Personal communication from PhD findings, UCL.

CHAIN: Combined Homeless Action and Information Network. (2009). *Street to Home, Annual report for London*, 1st April 2008–31st March 2009. London: CHAIN.

Davis, S., Greenish, W., Kennedy, P., and Jones, L. (2011). Supporting homeless people facing death with advanced liver disease. Report, Marie Curie Cancer Care and St Mungo's. www.mariecurie.org.uk; www.mungos.org.

Department of Health. (2008). *End of life Care Strategy: Promoting High Quality Care for Adults at the End of Life*. London: Department of Health.

Department of Health Office of the Chief Analyst. (2010). *Health Care for Single Homeless People 22 March*. London: Department of Health.

Homeless Link. (2009). Survey of Needs and Provision Report available at www.homeless.org.uk/snap-2009.

Kushel, M. and Miakowski, C. (2006). End of life care for homeless patients: 'She says she is there to help me in any situation'. *Journal of the American Medical Association,* **296**: 2959–66.

Mahony, S., McHenry, J., Snow, D., Cassin, C., Schumacher, D., and Selwyn, P. A. (2008). Review of barriers to utilization of the Medicare hospice benefits in urban populations and strategies for enhanced access. *Journal of Urban Health,* **85**(2): 281–90.

Moller, D. (2005). None left behind: Urban poverty, social experience, and re-thinking palliative care. *Journal of Palliative Medicine,* **8**(1): 17–19.

O'Connell, J. J. (2005). Premature mortality in homeless populations: A review of the literature. Nashville: National Health Care for the Homeless Council.

Podymow, T., Turnbull, J., and Coyle, D. (2006). Shelter-based palliative care for the homeless terminally ill. *Palliative Medicine,* **20**: 81–6.

Route to Success Series, found at www.endoflifecareforaults.nhs.uk, available from December 2010.

Song, J., Bartel, D., Ratner, E., Alderton, L., Hudson, B., and Ahluwalia, J. (2007). Dying on the streets: Homeless Persons' Concerns and Desires about End of Life Care. *Journal of General Internal Medicine,* **22**: 435–41.

Song, J., Wall, M., Ratner, E., Bartels, D., Ulvestad, N., and Gelberg, L. (2008). Engaging homeless persons in end of life preparations. *Journal of General Internal Medicine,* **23**(12): 2031–45.

Tarzian, A., Neal, M., and O'Neil, A. (2005). Attitudes, experiences, and beliefs affecting end of life decision making among homeless individuals. *Journal of Palliative Medicine,* **8**(1): 36–48.

Chapter 16

Travellers' and gypsies' death and dying

Regina McQuillan

Traveller Case History

JW, a 63-year-old man, presented with metastatic colorectal cancer. He was a Traveller, who lived in designated housing for Travellers. He was mainly settled but would travel by trailer during the summer, and also in November, when he would travel to his family graves, staying away from his house for a number of weeks at a time. He kept a trailer in the front garden. His wife was a Traveller; they had five adult children, all married and four of them living close to him.

Following his diagnosis, he was offered palliative chemotherapy. After his first course of chemotherapy, he was referred to the hospital palliative care team, and subsequently to the community palliative care team. He continued to attend hospital for chemotherapy. Despite an initial response, his health deteriorated. He, and more particularly his wife, appreciated the support of the community palliative care team for management of symptoms, education about medication, support for his children, and advice about how to support their grandchildren.

Acute deteriorations in his health led to his re-admission to hospital on two occasions as he and his family wished to prolong his life and were anxious to have what they perceived to be best care. The oncology team, following discussion with the palliative care team, recognized that JW would not want to go to the hospice and would wish for hospital admission in situations where other patients would feel confident to be cared for at home. Re-admission was usually through the emergency room. JW wished to be at home as much as possible; his wife and family wanted to facilitate this. As he was deteriorating, his wife began to consider him dying at home, including moving him into the trailer in the front garden, so that he died there rather than in the house, and that after his death the trailer could be moved away or burnt. However, on reflection, and with the support of the community team, his wife came to the conclusion that if she did something so counter to their culture as to have him die at home, she might find it hard to live with the unease of her wider family and community after his death.

JW continued to deteriorate although he never acknowledged that he was dying. He was admitted to hospital and died three days later. During his final hospital stay large numbers of his extended family visited him and comforted his wife. The family ensured their presence did not interfere with the work of the hospital or the care of other patients.

> The work of the hospital and community palliative care teams supported the patient and family, but also played an important role in educating the emergency room staff and oncology team about the important aspects of death and dying in Traveller culture.

Gypsies and Travellers form part of a world-wide group of people who have, or had, a nomadic way of life, though nomadism is difficult to maintain in contemporary Western societies. In Africa and Asia there is nomadism for agricultural and pastoral reasons, but in this chapter the focus is on European Gypsies and Travellers and the population is referred to as Gypsies and Travellers, unless reference is being made to specific groups.

The biggest group of Gypsies and Travellers are Romany of whom there are an estimated 12 million world wide, with over 100 different groups with different languages and customs. There is a move to recognize this heterogeneity in Roma studies (Tremlett, 2009). There is a long history of distrust and discrimination in relation to Travellers and Gypsies which has included attempts to suppress the culture, including prohibition of the use of Romany dress and language and the removal of children from Roma families to be brought up by others in various European countries over the centuries (Drakakis-Smith, 2007; Hajioff, 2000). There have been attempts to force assimilation into the majority culture, for example by the Commission on Itinerancy in Ireland in 1963. (Ni Shuinéar, 2004)

Gypsy and Traveller societies can be considered collectivist rather than individualist. Collectivist societies value the needs of the family as much, if not more so, than the needs of the individual. Families are interconnected and the immediate family can include extended family such as aunts, uncles, and distant cousins. The strong emphasis on the importance of families attending life rituals means that there are large family gatherings, which can cause anxiety for the majority population if, for example, hundreds of people arrive in a town for funerals, weddings, or other family events. Other aspects of Traveller culture, including lack of formal employment, trading at fairs, and camping at unofficial sites, create hostility and tensions.

Gypsies and Travellers sometimes hide their identity so they can access things they believe may be denied to them if their ethnic origin was clear. In Ireland, this is called 'passing off', and parents reported that their children changed their accent or dress in certain situations to hide their identity (Our Geels, 2010). Vivian and Dundes (1986) report that American Roma in the US may identify themselves as Romanian, Native American, or Mexican to avoid Roma stereotyping.

In the UK, two groups, Romany Gypsies and Irish Travellers, are recognized as ethnic minorities by the Race Relations Act. The Office of the Deputy Prime Minister defined Gypsies and Travellers as 'persons of nomadic habit of life whatever their race or origin including such persons who on grounds only of their own or their family's or dependents' education or health needs or old age have ceased to travel temporarily or permanently but excluding members of an organised group of travelling show people or circus people travelling together as such' (Drakakis-Smith, 2007). This recognizes that an individual may be a Traveller or Gypsy, even if they are not mobile. The recent

NHS Primary Care Service Framework for Gypsies and Travellers has been developed for Romany Gypsies, Roma and Irish Travellers but also recognizes a number of other groups including Scottish Travellers, Welsh Gypsies, Bargees, Circus and Showground people, and New Travellers. Gypsies and Travellers are not enumerated separately in the census in the UK, but there are approximately 300,000 Gypsies and Travellers in Britain (Parry et al., 2007).

In Ireland, Travellers are recognized by the government as a separate group and are specifically named in discrimination legislation (Employment Equality Act 1998, Equal Status Act 2000). The All Ireland Health Traveller Study (Our Geels, 2010) undertook a census, and there are over 36,000 travellers in the Republic of Ireland and nearly 4,000 in Northern Ireland. The origin of Irish Travellers is not clear; there are suggestions that they are completely separate to the Irish population; other suggestions are that they are descended from dispossessed Irish who had been made landless during invasions. Travellers identify themselves and are identified by settled people as different to each other. Genetic studies suggest that the Traveller population is endogenous rather than as a result of migration eg of Roma into Ireland (North et al., 2000; Murphy et al., 1999).

Gypsy and Traveller health

Much focus of health research among these populations has been on genetics (50%); infectious disease (12%) and health service use (22%) (Zeman et al., 2003). Hajioff and McKee (2000) consider that the research sometimes shows a greater concern for the majority population than the Roma population.

Gypsies and Travellers have poorer health than other populations. Life expectancy for Roma people is 6 years less than the majority population in Bulgaria; 11 years less for Roma men and 14 years less for Roma women in the Czech Republic; and 13 years less for men and 17 years less for women in Slovakia (Sepkowitz, 2006). The All Ireland Traveller Health Study (Our Geels, 2010) shows that the average life expectancy of a Traveller man is 62 compared to 77 years for a settled man, and of a Traveller woman is 70, compared to a settled woman which is 81 years. The life expectancy of Traveller men has not improved since 1987, and the gap in life expectancy of Traveller men and settled men has widened. Respiratory illnesses in men and women, and external causes (accidents, suicide, poisoning, including alcohol and drugs) in men lead to most excess of deaths.

A review of the health of Gypsies and Travellers in England (Peters et al., 2009) showed poorer health than age- and sex-matched controls from deprived areas and ethnic minority populations. Respiratory illnesses were particularly prevalent; there were no differences between Gypsies and Travellers and the matched populations for cancer, stroke, and diabetes.

Gypsies and Travellers and health service use

In Peters' (2009) study, 69% of Gypsies and Travellers were registered with GPs compared to 96% of the matched population. In both the Republic of Ireland (ROI) and

Northern Ireland (NI), approximately 90% of Travellers got their health information from their GP (Our Geels, 2010). However, Travellers in Ireland are more than twice as likely to use the Accident and Emergency Department as the settled population. Travellers are more likely to be admitted via the emergency room than electively (80% vs 35%), are less likely to have a discharge letter written (67% vs 100%), were less likely to have outpatient clinic follow up appointments (40% vs 77%) or to be referred to clinical support services (21% vs 62%) in comparison to the settled population (Traveller Health Unit, 2004). Travellers are less likely to have complete trust in health care professionals (41% in ROI, 34.6% in NI) compared to 82.7% in the settled population.

Irish Travellers are likely to use healers, and also to use faith- or religion-based healing. Faith healing includes visiting places associated with healing, such as Knock in Ireland and Lourdes in France, or holy wells, and the use of objects such as relics of saints, etc. There is great respect for clergy and specific prayers, including masses, are often requested for the patient (McQuillan and Van Doorsaler, 2007).

Vivian and Dundes (2004) published a review of Roma culture and health in the US which is based on case studies and individual reports. They report that it is important for Roma to avoid contamination of what is pure by what is less pure. Roma believe that the lower half of the body is less pure than the upper half. This is part of the reason why Romany women wear long skirts. Roma believe that something which touches the lower body, including soap and wash cloths, should not touch the upper body. Health care workers should wash their hands or change gloves if they move from examining the lower body to the upper body.

Hospice and palliative care and end of life care

Little research has been carried out among Gypsy and Traveller populations worldwide about hospice or end of life care. Vivian and Dundes (2004) report that the presence of the family is very important for Roma at times of serious illness; up to a hundred people may accompany a patient. Roma believe that after death the soul retraces its steps for one year and for that reason the body needs to be intact; organ donation is not appropriate. Grief at the time of death can be very demonstrative, with screaming and crying. There are traditions carried out, including the lighting of candles and asking the dead person for forgiveness, and it is important for the bereaved that these are carried out.

Van Cleemput et al. (2007), as part of a qualitative study on health-related beliefs and experiences, carried out semi-structured interviews with 27 Gypsies and Travellers in England. The respondents had a fatalistic attitude, with expectations of poor health. There was an exceptionally strong aversion to discussing cancer and a fear of death and dying.

Research undertaken by McQuillan and Van Doorsaler (2007) in Ireland explored the views of Travellers of hospice and palliative care. Travellers had little knowledge of hospice and palliative care. They were fearful of discussing cancer. The word was avoided or when mentioned was accompanied by prayers or blessings. The belief expressed was that by discussing cancer or other serious illnesses, bad luck would befall the speakers.

When a Traveller is seriously ill it is the custom from extended family and friends to visit and spend time supporting the patient and the immediate family. Travellers consider the habits of settled people, whereby only small numbers of people visit, inappropriate. Traveller custom can mean that large crowds would wish to visit, especially as the patient is approaching death. Travellers are often demonstrative and the combination of demonstrative behaviour and large crowds can lead to staff in hospitals or hospices feeling overwhelmed. Unless staff understand the importance of this behaviour, staff responses, which can include restriction of visiting and calling security, can increase distress. Identifying key people within the family and using clergy can facilitate Travellers visiting and the management of institutional concerns.

When a patient is dying families will often request a priest to attend for prayers and blessings. Items of religious significance such as medals or relics may be placed around the patient and at times placed over the affected area of the body. Staff need to ensure they are not lost during medical and nursing care.

Hospitals are seen as places of hope, where cure is possible. Hospices are seen as a last resort, and although Travellers who had experienced hospice care were positive about the experience, it was not an experience that was welcomed, being considered recognition and acceptance of the terminal nature of an illness.

Travellers were more positive toward community palliative care as a way of providing support for the patient and family. Many respondents saw advantages to the person being cared for at home, but death at home was usually considered unacceptable. This is because of the feelings of great sadness associated with the death, which can mean that families find it hard to stay in a place where a death has occurred. Traditionally the trailer of a person who dies, especially if the death happened in the trailer, would be burned. Families would move away from the site. This happens less frequently now, partly for economic reasons and also because more Travellers live in houses. More commonly now, families may try to sell a trailer associated with someone who dies, but it can be difficult to find a buyer for a trailer in which a death has occurred. Travellers who live in houses may, following a death, move out of the house for a period of time, and not return until the house has been redecorated and blessed. For these reasons, Travellers usually do not want to die at home.

Research carried out by the Parish of the Travelling People (Brack and Monaghan, 2007), although limited in its scope, echoed results found by McQuillan and Van Doorsaler. This included the fear of serious illness and of death, strong religious beliefs and expression, including the importance of religious rituals to support the sick, the centrality of the family, and the importance of visiting the sick. Travellers also reported the importance of being present if something were to go wrong, that the sick person be surrounded by 'their own', and that the sick person have the opportunity to pass on their last wishes.

After death

For many Irish Travellers having an elaborate coffin and headstone is considered a sign of love and respect and families may go into debt to pay for a funeral. In Ireland the deceased is often buried within two or three days of death, and if mourners do not arrive in time to view the remains a request may be made that the coffin be opened in the church so they may pay their respects; this may cause anxiety for clergy or undertakers, but this can be very important for the bereaved (Brack and Monaghan, 2007).

Traditionally, Travellers are buried in the burial ground associated with their family. Nowadays, especially as more Travellers are settled rather than nomadic, Travellers may be buried where their family live. There can be tension in the family if there are different views between the family of origin and the family of marriage about the place of burial, and negotiation is needed. Given that many hundreds of people will attend funerals and that it is usual for there to be loud and demonstrative expression of grief, Traveller funerals can cause stress for the settled population. This can lead to intervention by the police which, if not appropriately handled, can increase tensions.

Bereavement

A number of studies emphasize the grief and sense of loss experienced when a member of the community dies. This can be so extreme among Irish Travellers as to cause the family to move away from the place of death or burn the trailer, as outlined above. The use of alcohol to cope with bereavement was recognized as not always being helpful (McQuillan and Van Doorsaler, 2007; Van Cleemput et al., 2007; Brack and Monaghan, 2007).

Conclusion

Travellers and Gypsies are a diverse population characterized in this context as being a collectivist society, with strong emphasis on the importance of family. This means that it would not be unusual for a hundred people to wish to visit a patient. Travellers and Gypsies have experienced discrimination for centuries which can lead to distrust by these populations of the majority population. They have poorer health and shorter life expectancy than the majority population, are fearful of serious illness and death, and avoid discussing serious illness, especially cancer and dying. Irish Travellers are reluctant to be admitted to hospices as this is a recognition of death. Irish Travellers are also unlikely to want to die at home, because of the loneliness associated with a place of death. Reluctance to engage with hospice and palliative care, combined with the large crowds accompanying a patient and family during illness and bereavement, can mean that caring for Travellers and Gypsies can be challenging. Identifying key people in the family or support network, recognizing the need for clear explanations, and recognizing the differences between different families can all help health care staff and the Travellers and Gypsies cope.

Resources

- www.gypsy-traveller.org
- www.nationalgypsytravellerfederation.org
- www.paveepoint.ie
- The full report of the research carried out by Regina McQuillan and Onje Van Doorsaler is available at www.sfh.ie, under publications.

References

Brack, J. and Monaghan, S. (2007). *Travellers' Last Rites: Responding to Death in a Cultural Context*. Dublin: Parish of the Travelling People.

Drakakis-Smith, A. (2007). Nomadism: A moving myth? Policies of exclusion and the Gypsy/Traveller response. *Mobilities*, **2**(3): 463–87.

Employment Equality Act 1998. www.irishstatutebook.ie/ZZA21Y1998.html (accessed 1 Dec. 2010).

Equal Status Act 2000. www.irishstatutebook.ie/ZZA8Y2000.l (accessed 1 Dec. 2010).

Hajioff, S. and McKee, M. (2000). The Health of the Roma people: A review of the published literature. *Journal of Epidemiology and Community Health*, **54**: 864–9.

Ireland, Adelaide and Meath Hospital incorporating the National Children's Hospital (AMNCH). (2005). Use of hospital facilities by the Traveller community. Kildare, Traveller Health Unit in the Eastern Region. Available at: http://www.paveepoint.ie/pdf/TallaghtHospital.pdf (accessed 29 Oct. 2010).

McQuillan, R. and Van Doorsaler, O. (2007). Indigenous ethnic minorities and palliative care: Exploring the views of Irish Travellers and palliative care staff. *Palliative Medicine*, **21**(7): 635–41.

Murphy, M., McHugh, B., Tighe, O., Mayne, P., O'Neill, C., Naughten, E., and Croke, D. T. (1999). Genetic basis of transferase-deficient galactosaemia in Ireland and the population history of the Irish Travellers. *European Journal of Human Genetics*, **7**: 549–54.

Ní Shuinéar, S. (2004). Apocrypha to canon: Inventing Irish Traveller history. *History Ireland*, **12**(4): 15–19.

North, K. E., Martin, L. J., and Crawford, M. H. (2000). The origins of the Irish Travellers and the genetic structure of Ireland. *Annals of Human Biology*, **27**(5): 453–65.

Our Geels. (2010). All Ireland Traveller Health Study. School of Public Health, Physiotherapy and Population Science, University College Dublin.

Parry, G., Van Cleemput, P., Peters, J., Walters, S., Thomas, K., and Cooper, C. (2007). Health status of Gypsies and Travellers in England. *Journal of Epidemiology and Community Health*, **61**: 198–204.

Peters, J., Parry, G. D., Van Cleemput, P., Moore, J., Cooper, C. L., and Walters, S. (2009). Health and the use of health services: A comparison between Gypsies and Travellers and other ethnic groups. *Ethnicity and Health*, **14**(4): 359–77.

Sepkowitz, K. (2006). Health of the world's Roma population. *The Lancet*, **367**: 1707–8.

Tremlett, A, (2009). Bringing hybridity to heterogeneity in Romani Studies. *Romani Studies*, **19**(2): 147–68.

Van Cleemput, P., Glenys, P., Thomas, K., Peters, J., and Cooper, C. (2007). Health related beliefs and experiences of Gypsies and Travellers: A qualitative study. *Journal of Epidemiology and Community Health*, **61**(3): 205–10.

Vivian, C. and Dundes, L. (2004). The crossroads of culture and health among the Roma (Gypsies). *Journal of Nursing Scholarship*, **36**(1): 86–91.

Zeman, C. L., Depken, D. E., and Senchina, D. S. (2003). Roma health issues: A review of the literature and discussion. *Ethnicity & Health*, **8**(3): 223–49.

Chapter 17

Asylum seekers and refugees

Nigel G. J. Dodds

This chapter aims to highlight the distinct needs of asylum seekers and refugees. Despite sharing a label given by the international community distinguishing these groups from others in this book, asylum seekers and refugees are not a homogenous group and as individuals do not necessarily share a similar set of clearly defined needs. There is a wealth of literature on the needs and experiences of these groups, yet not in relation to palliative care (Blanche and Endersby, 2004). Throughout history, societies have failed to meet the challenges of ensuring that those seeking refuge have safe passage and secure resettlement. The constant presence of conflict and the persecution of individuals and groups mean that there remains a flow of enforced migration from one country to another. Health and social care systems continue to evolve within complex social and political contexts. Asylum seekers and refugees remain high on the agenda of political and media debate, and those responsible for providing health and social care have a considerable challenge in attempting to ensure that they can access appropriate services. Whilst not excluded by law, it is clear that asylum seekers and refugees continue to experience some degree of social exclusion (Cabinet Office, 2010). There is evidence that members of all ethnic minority groups are rarely afforded the access to specialist palliative care that they require (Koffman et al., 2007). Additionally, explicit and less obvious racism can result in inequalities for black and ethnic minority groups in the health care system and is likely to impact on their experience of health care (Szczepura, 2005).

Asylum seekers and refugees—contemporary definitions, understandings, and legal context

Globally, estimates vary greatly about the numbers of people who are identified as asylum seekers or refugees. Varying definitions of these groups hamper accurate data collection. Despite this the United Nations High Commissioner for Refugees (2009) estimated that globally there were 36,464,160 persons of concern to the organization, and half of these were thought to be children.

In the United Kingdom in 2009, the number of asylum applications was seen to be at its lowest in 16 years with 24,250 principal applicants making asylum claims (Refugee Council, 2009). Of this group the Refugee Council supported around 1,000 unaccompanied children (Refugee Council, 2010). The greatest numbers of people seeking refuge in the United Kingdom currently are from Afghanistan, Iran, China, Iraq, and Eritrea (Culley and Dyson, 2010). Asylum applications only accounted for 4% of the UK's total immigration figure in 2007 (Centre for Social Justice, 2008). Independent research commissioned by the Refugee Council on decisions made by asylum seekers who come to the UK has also shown that more than two-thirds did not specifically choose to come to the UK. The decision over destination was often made by the agents who facilitated the journey and access to travel documents (Crawley, 2010). Europe looks after 14% of all refugees and asylum seekers, and the United Kingdom is home to less than 2% of the total figure. In Europe the numbers of people seeking asylum who are granted refugee status varies greatly, from 3% in Slovenia, to 77% in Finland (Refugee Council, 2009).

Asylum seekers and refugees are frequently cited in the wider debate on general immigration issues. The terms 'asylum', 'asylum seeker', and 'refugee' are often mis-interpreted or used interchangeably. It is hardly surprising that the misunderstand-ings surrounding these terms may give rise to confusion, fear, and resultant prejudice and discrimination towards asylum seekers and refugees from the general public and health care providers. Whilst the media is often criticised for such misunderstandings, there is a long history of prejudice and discrimination across the globe towards these groups. Reporting on asylum issues regularly fails to distinguish between economic migrants and asylum seekers or refugees; statistics are often unsourced, exaggerated, or unexplained (ICAR, 2005).

In the United Kingdom an asylum seeker is defined as a person who has submitted an application for protection under the Geneva Convention, and is waiting for the claim to be decided by the Home Office. A refugee is a person who has been accepted under the Geneva Convention, and has been granted Indefinite Leave to Remain (ILR), and therefore has permanent residence in the United Kingdom. Some asylum seekers may be granted Exceptional Leave to Enter or Remain (ELE or ELR). Here the Home Office accepts that currently the person cannot return to their home country. ELR gives the individual the right to stay for four years. He or she is then expected to return home if the situation in their country of origin improves. To claim asylum and go on to be recognized as a refugee, an individual must have left their country of origin and be unable to return because they have a well-founded fear of persecution because of their race; religion; nationality; political opinion; or membership of a particular social group (UNHCR, 1951).

The vast majority of all those seeking asylum do so in countries neighbouring their own. Over half a million refugees have fled wartorn Sudan to neighbouring countries, yet only 265 Sudanese people applied for asylum in the UK in 2008 (Refugee Council, 2009). Those who travel to wealthier nations such as the UK and the US need access to significant resources to enable their passage.

Access to health care and palliative care

Asylum seekers arriving in the UK or any other host nation may have a very limited knowledge of the health care and welfare systems of that nation (Crawley, 2010). Arriving in a new country and even once established as a refugee, these individuals are likely to experience poverty, dependence, and a lack of cohesive social support. Children and elderly people may be living in fragmented families, or with people who are unfamiliar to them. They may have experienced the death of close family members, or be unaware of their current circumstances, leading to an increased sense of vulnerability (Connelly et al., 2006). Such factors can undermine both physical and mental health. Arriving in another country, the asylum seeker or refugee who is faced with a life threatening illness is likely to have the same basic physical health needs as anyone else. But on top of these basic health needs the asylum seeker is likely to face a restrictive, complex, and overloaded asylum system in an alien society and psychological distress is widespread (Burnett and Peel, 2001).

Many asylum seekers and refugees have major health problems that may require palliative care. The numbers of individuals from sub-Saharan Africa affected by HIV and AIDS is enormous and has had devastating consequences on the continent. Despite advances in the treatment of HIV disease many asylum seekers and refugees present late with disease and not having had access to highly active anti-retroviral therapy (HAART) due to not knowing their HIV status or inability to access such medicines. They may not declare their HIV status to officials in their new country, fearing prejudice or deportation (Easterbrook and Meadway, 2001). There is growing evidence of a rising problem amongst women who have been 'trafficked' as sex workers to another country. With increasing numbers of women with HIV and AIDS and cervical cancer secondary to sexually transmitted infections (Zimmerman et al., 2009). This group may seek asylum having been arrested by authorities or having escaped from their persecutors. They may also present late with disease and need urgent access to palliative care.

The equitable provision of health care to asylum seekers and refugees requires the application of the consistent principle that the person is treated as an individual, as 'the terms refugee and asylum seeker denote a situation rather than an identity' (Burnett and Fassil, 2002: 8). In the UK, all asylum seekers, refugees, and their dependants have the right to free health care. However the capacity of local services to provide for these vulnerable groups can be limited. Although perhaps not deliberately, these groups are often excluded due to society's failure to meet their specific needs (Koffman and Camps, 2008). In the UK, asylum seekers will be given housing and minimal finances to provide for basic needs. However asylum seekers are not permitted to work and are not able to claim any supplementary state welfare benefits such as illness benefits or funeral expenses (UK Border Agency, 2010). Poverty is a real issue further stigmatizing and erecting barriers to accessing appropriate health care support.

Like other minority groups in society, asylum seekers and refugees have an increased likelihood of dying in hospital (Koffman et al., 2007). It is recognized that these groups may have a lower awareness of health care services in general (Burnett and Peel, 2001) that may limit their use of palliative care services. Some health care professionals may not refer minority groups such as asylum seekers and refugees to palliative care providers because of a perception that they may be Christian based organizations, and inappropriate for individuals from different cultural backgrounds (Johnson, 2009). Furthermore refugees and asylum seekers may perceive service providers to be untrustworthy, inflexible to their needs and be concerned that palliative care professionals may have negative attitudes towards them (Krakauer and Crenner, 2002).

On making telephone contact with Kim, a refugee from North Korea, he appeared extremely anxious about being seen by the community palliative care team in his home.

This caused some difficulties for the team who were used to seeing patients in their homes. A team discussion highlighted that he might be fearful of authorities due to experiences in his home country. Following an initial meeting in the outpatient clinic at the hospice, Kim informed his nurse that he had been visited by police several times before he fled his country and tortured in his own home.

A further barrier that exists to the access of health care and palliative care concerns those asylum seekers and refugees held in detention centres. The United Kingdom has the largest number of places to detain this group, with the capacity to detain 3,100 individuals at any one time. Despite international legislation and UK Home Office guidelines, 2,000 children are held in UK detention centres each year (McCarthy, 2010). Detainees may be victims of torture, trafficking, and have serious mental health problems. Those with health needs related to chronic diseases such as HIV/AIDS and cancer are unlikely to have them met (Aspinall and Watters, 2010). There is a dearth of evidence on palliative care provision for asylum seekers and refugees held in detention centres, but the lack of a basic level of health care is astonishing given the needs of these individuals.

Language

Health care professionals may lack awareness, skills, and training to help the most excluded groups (Cabinet Office, 2010). A study undertaken by the British Medical Association (2004) exploring General Practitioners' experiences of providing primary care to these groups highlights a number of challenges. Interpreted consultations frequently take longer. Language differences require interpreting services and the translation of key documents relating to health care all of which may be thought to impact on the services given to the host populations. Having complex needs and different lifestyles, can add to the difficulty of accessing services. These groups may also have different aspirations and expectations of health and social care services, and users can feel 'invisible' or discriminated against when using the services (Cabinet Office, 2010).

Alketa, an elderly Kosovan refugee, spoke no English and lived with her family. The family, all of whom spoke English, did not want to use interpreting services in meetings with health care professionals. This initially caused some degree of conflict between the family and the palliative care team. However the palliative care team persisted in their requests to use an interpreter thus enabling an impartial interpreter for consultations. Alketa was then involved in a conversation about advance care planning which ultimately led to her choosing her place of death.

Culture

Individuals from other countries are likely to have varying cultures to those of their adopted homeland. Culture is far more than language and is likely to determine individuals' explanatory model of health and illness, affecting the way they perceive disease and its causes, as well as its treatments. Behaviour towards health and illness and perceptions of health care professionals may not match those of the host nation (Helman, 2007). Health care services must be culturally competent.

A refugee from Zimbabwe who was receiving care from a hospice stated that he welcomed the image of a world map in the hospice reception that indicated the joint working between this hospice and a hospice in his home country. He felt that this acknowledged a link between this country and his homeland and made him feel more accepted in the building.

Many asylum seekers and refugees will have been subjected to oppressive conditions and torture in their country of departure (Culley and Dyson, 2010). Whilst the physical impact of, for example, war, torture, rape, assault, trafficking, landmine injuries, and malnutrition will lead to specific physical health problems, there is also a psychological impact that may lead to feelings of fear of those in authority in the new country (Blanche and Endersby, 2004). Whilst 1 in 6 refugees has a severe physical health problem, two-thirds appear to have experienced anxiety and depression (Burnett and Peel, 2001). Individuals may display signs of depression and anxiety, panic attacks and agoraphobia, which are often exacerbated by social isolation and poverty. The particular expressions of fear and mental health problems may not 'fit' with palliative care providers' normal understanding of these issues. Mental illness is defined within a given culture, that is the group defines what is normal and that which is abnormal. 'Normal' rules of defining and understanding mental illness may not apply for refugees and asylum seekers (Helman, 2007). Specialist help may be required to understand cultural frameworks.

Women and older people

Asma, a 60-year-old woman from Iraq, had ELR refugee status, with two years left of her permission to remain in the UK. She was admitted to her local acute hospital and found to have advanced cervical cancer. Sheltered by and financially supported by relatives living in the UK, Asma had maintained a low profile since developing symptoms of illness. She had feared that presenting with symptoms earlier in her disease may have led to early deportation. By the time she sought help, her advanced disease excluded her from any active treatment. She was seen by the hospital palliative care team who addressed immediate symptom control issues. Asma was not registered with a General Practitioner, and was anxious about being referred to her local community palliative care team in case they were in some way connected to authorities who might deport her. With this patient, the priority was to develop a trusting relationship and ensure she understood that being known to a General Practitioner and palliative care team would not lead to any involvement from government authorities.

Older asylum seekers and refugees, especially women are thought to have particular problems in accessing health services. This group may be resistant to approaching authorities and public bodies due to experiences of being persecuted, trafficked, or discriminated against. They may be more vulnerable due to their reliance on their persecutors or younger generations for access to health care (Connelly et al., 2006). Women and older people may be especially fearful of services due to their vulnerability and history of rape, assault, and sexual harassment. Women and older people are less likely to be English speaking and this may increase fear of service providers (Connelly et al., 2006). Clear policies of non-discrimination need to be espoused and taught to enable the clear communication of open access to these groups.

Practice challenge

*Mohammed was a man in his early forties from Sierra Leone with a refugee status of
Indefinite Leave to Remain in the UK. He was living in South London when he was
referred to the community palliative care team following an admission to his local acute
hospital, where he had been diagnosed with a rare form of metastatic cancer of the gall
bladder. He was referred for support with pain control. However he was noted to be frail
and in need of general support in the community as he was relatively isolated.*

*Mohammed lived in small flat on a large housing estate with his nephew. They had
little access to money other than for basic provisions. Mohammed made it clear to the
nurse initially visiting him at home that if there was no medical treatment to help him
he wished to return to his homeland. However at a follow-up hospital appointment
Mohammed was advised by his oncology team that chemotherapy may help him, believing this could lengthen Mohammed's life. Mohammed reported back to his nurse his
expectation that this treatment would cure him. As the time for Mohammed's treatment drew nearer he became frailer. The palliative care team attempted to discuss the
reality of the situation with Mohammed. However he remained clear that he wished to
have chemotherapy. Mohammed had clearly expressed his wish to return home to die
but was aiming for a cure for his cancer. With Mohammed's permission the palliative
care nurse visiting him at home spoke with the hospital palliative care team. It was
agreed that the hospital palliative care nurse would attend Mohammed's next oncology
appointment with him. At this appointment the nurse was able to support Mohammed
in discussions with the oncologist and the oncologist, was able to understand
Mohammed's wish to return home if he was dying, his frailty, and low level of social
support at home. A clear consultation took place. It was decided that Mohammed
would not receive chemotherapy. With financial support from his brother who lived in
the USA, Mohammed made a prompt decision to return to his hometown in Sierra
Leone where he died a month after his return with his family around him. For
Mohammed, being at home equated to a good death.*

This case study highlights the need for joint working across sectors and the importance
of avoiding assumptions. The community palliative care team were able to shed light on
Mohammed's home situation, his goals, and expectations. Communicating this to colleagues in the acute sector enabled honest discussions to take place that led to Mohammed
making decisions about his future care and preferred place of death. Had Mohammed
not been enabled to make a more informed decision he may have gone on to have chemotherapy and remained much weaker and too frail to return home to Sierra Leone.

This chapter has provided some background to the general issues facing asylum
seekers and refugees. Clearly more needs to be done to ensure that these individuals
have equitable access to palliative care. More detailed research on their needs and how
to meet these in relation to end of life care is urgently required.

Resources

- Refugee Council: www.refugeecouncil.org.uk/
- United Nations Refugee Agency: -www.unhcr.org.uk/
- Refugees International: -www.refintl.org/

References

Aspinall, P. and Watters, C. (2010). Refugees and asylum seekers: A review from an equality and human rights perspective. [Online] Available at: www.equalityhumanrights.com/uploaded_files/research/refugees_and_asylum_seekers_research_report.pdf. Accessed 20 Oct. 2010.

Blanche, M. and Endersby, C. (2004). Refugees. In D. Oliviere and B. Monroe (eds), *Death, Dying and Social Differences*. Oxford: Oxford University Press.

British Medical Association. (2004). *Meeting the Healthcare Needs of Refugees and Asylum Seekers—A Survey of General Practitioners*. London: British Medical Association.

Burnett, A. and Fassil, Y. (2002). *Meeting the Health Needs of Refugee and Asylum Seekers in the UK: An Information and Resource Pack for Health Workers*. London: Department of Health.

Burnett, A. and Peel, M. (2001). Asylum seekers and refugees in Britain: Health needs of asylum seekers and refugees. *BMJ*, **322**(7285): 544–47.

Cabinet Office. (2010). *Inclusion Health: Improving the Way We Meet the Primary Health Care Needs of the Socially Excluded*. London: HM Government.

Connelly, N., Forsythe, L. A., Njike, G., and Rudiger, A. (2006). *Older Refugees in the UK: A Literature Review*. London: Age Concern and Refugee Council.

Crawley, H. (2010). *Chance or Choice? Understanding Why Asylum Seekers Come to the UK*. London: The Refugee Council.

Culley, L. and Dyson, S. (2010). *Ethnicity and Healthcare Practice: A Guide for the Primary Care Team*. London: Quay Books.

Easterbrook, P. and Meadway, J. (2001). The changing epidemiology of HIV infection: New challenges for HIV palliative care. *Journal of the Royal Society of Medicine*, **94**: 442–8.

Helman, C. G. (2007). *Culture, Health and Illness*, 5th edn. London: Hodder and Arnold.

Information Centre about Asylum Seekers and Refugees. (2005). Key issues: Public opinion on asylum and refugee issues. Briefing June 2005. London: ICAR. www.icar.org.uk/download.php?id=263.

Johnson, M. R. D. (2009). End of life care in ethnic minorities. *BMJ*, **338**: 489–90.

Koffman, J., Burke, G., Dias, A., Ravel, B., Byrne, J., Gonzales, J., et al. (2007). Demographic factors and awareness of palliative care and related services. *Palliative Medicine*, **21**(2): 145–53.

Koffman, J. and Camps, M. (2008). No way in: Including disadvantaged population and patient groups at the end of life. In S. Payne, et al. (eds), *Palliative Care Nursing: Principles and Evidence for Practice*, 2nd edn. Maidenhead, UK: Open University Press.

Krakauer, E. L. and Crenner, C. (2002). Barriers to optimum end-of-life care for minority patients. *Journal of the American Geriatrics Society*, **50**(1): 182–90.

McCarthy, M. (2010). Out of sight? *BMJ*, **341**: 326–7.

Refugee Council. (2009). *Tell It Like It Is: The Truth About Asylum*. London: Refugee Council.

Refugee Council. (2010). *Refugee Council Briefing August 2010: Recent Developments Relating to the Plans to Return Unaccompanied Children to Afghanistan*. London: Refugee Council.

Szczepura, A. (2005). Access to health care for ethnic minority populations. *Post Graduate Medical Journal*, **81**(953): 141–7.

UK Border Agency. (2010). Asylum support [online]. Available at: www.ukba.homeoffice.gov.uk/asylum/support/. Accessed 23 Oct. 2010.

United Nations High Commissioner for Refugees. (1951). *Convention and Protocol Relating the Status of Refugees*. Geneva: UNHCR.

United Nations High Commissioner for Refugees. (2009). New threats, new challenges: Global report 2009 [online]. Available at: www.unhcr.org/4c08f27d9.pdf. Accessed 30 Sept. 2010.

Zimmerman, C., Oram, S., and Watts, C. (2009). Meeting the health needs of trafficked persons. *BMJ*, **339**: 642–3.

Chapter 18

Palliative care for substance misusers

Chris Farnham

The case for studying this group

There is a growing awareness that palliative care as defined by the WHO (2004) is applicable as a practice to many more fields than had previously been recognized. Services now see patients with a wide variety of diagnoses and from a widening spectrum of society bringing a new set of palliative challenges. These challenges can present both pharmacologically and organizationally. This chapter will explore the evidence and practice of working with patients who have a substance misuse history and try to explore the specific palliative care needs of this group. Substances that are misused are many and varied and vary between countries and continents. Much of the research in this field comes specifically from a North American context and ignores emerging nations. It might be argued that as societies become more industrialized, so the influx of substances misused will change to mirror those seen in Western societies. There is little in the way of evidence based practice for palliative care and its use and delivery to this group.

What is the problem?

Recent data from the UK National Drug Treatment Monitoring System (October 2010) suggests that 206,889 individuals aged 18 and over were recorded as in contact with structured drug treatment services in England for 2009/10 and most clients in contact with treatment were using opiates and/or crack cocaine (84%). Cannabis was used as a primary drug by 7% of clients and powder cocaine as a primary drug by 5% of clients.

The British Crime Survey (2010) found that one third of 15–59 year olds have used illegal drugs at some point and 6% use them regularly (Hoare et al., 2010). All data shows that this is not unique to the UK and is similar in all developed nations. The vast majority of substance misusers are not in treatment programmes however and this might be the tip of the iceberg. The common misconception of the homeless drug user is as outmoded and incorrect as misconceptions about HIV and its sufferers were in the 1980s. It is for this reason that new thinking in our education of health professionals should include a questioning of all clients about drug use, be they homeless or city lawyers.

As time goes on it is not only the numbers of users that change but also the drugs taken. The British Crime Survey from the Home Office for 2009/10 offers an estimate of illicit drug use in adults aged between 16–59 for England and Wales (Hoare and Moon, 2010). It suggests that 8.6% of adults used illicit drugs and 3.1% had used a class A drug in the past year. It also estimates that 3.3% of adults were frequent drug users (using a drug more than once a month on average in the last year), where cannabis was the most commonly used drug, followed by powder cocaine. A Home Office publication, 'Seizures of Drugs in England and Wales, 2009/2010', showed that the number of drug seizures made in this time period had nearly doubled since 2004 (Mulchandani et al., 2010). New 'legal highs' such as mephadrone emerged only to be legislated against in April 2010. However as soon as one drug is contained new ones are developed such as NRG-1 or naphrone or old ones resurrected such as MDAI, an antidepressant. London has approximately 75,000 'problem' drug users and for them the cost of drug taking has dropped remarkably. Cocaine now comes in 'basic' or 'luxury' levels depending on the quality of the product.

Case history

Annie was a 32-year-old woman living in a hostel in central London. She was referred to a hospice as she had metastatic carcinoma of the cervix, with lung and bone disease. She had a long history of opioid drug use and alcohol dependency as well as a personality disorder. She had had multiple custodial sentences.

Her main problems on referral were pain and a vaginal fistula. These were causing the hostel staff problems as she became more bed bound and unable to wash herself. Her pain relief became a problem as other hostel users understood the nature of her analgesic regime. This carried the risk that other users might want to appropriate her opioids.

Annie was seen and assessed by a palliative community specialist nurse and doctor together with her case worker. She identified that she wanted to stay in the hostel, being aware that she would probably die soon.

She and the team signed a contract whereby her general practitioner was to be her sole prescriber and stating that she would be managed with pain killing patches and a very limited supply of breakthrough painkillers that would be monitored regularly by her nurses.

The hostel staff were offered education and support in helping to care for a dying person and community nurses visited daily to help with dressing changes. Equipment and a hospital bed were put into the hostel by the occupational therapist and specialist palliative care social workers offered counseling and benefits advice.

The out of hours services, including the London Ambulance Service and doctors, were alerted to the fact that she wanted to stay at the hostel and she died there eighteen days after referral. The hostel staff were supported by the hospice bereavement service.

What is dependency?

This is a term that was first used by Edwards and Gross (1976). It has been much modified over the years and is well integrated into ICD-10 and DSM 1V. It involves the following:

◆ Primacy of drug-seeking behaviour
◆ Increased tolerance

◆ Signs of withdrawal

◆ Continued taking of substances despite evidence of harm

◆ Rapid reinstatement after abstinence

◆ Narrowing of the drug-taking repertoire

◆ Loss of control

◆ Aberrant drug-taking to avoid withdrawal.

Why do this group need palliative care?

In 2004 the World Health Organization defined four main areas where substance misuse impacted on the health economy:

◆ Chronic Health Effects i.e. liver cirrhosis

◆ Acute Health Effects i.e. overdose and injuries

◆ Acute Social Problems i.e. arrest and family breakdown

◆ Chronic Social Problems i.e. loss of employment and low income

We know that substance misusers have higher associated health problems such as viral-borne diseases as shown by Gough and colleagues (2010) in their systematic review of the rates of HIV and Hepatitis in high and low risk groups in the USA. However this is only a small snapshot of their problems. Many are homeless, have cardiovascular risk factors and are poor at accessing statutory health services. As a consequence of some of these factors they have a higher death rate than their non using equivalents. Studies from the 1980s onwards have focused on HIV and it is estimated that in 2008 there were 2.7 million new infections. Deaths from HIV peaked at 2.2 million in 2004 with an estimated 2 million deaths in 2008 (UNAIDS annual report, 2009). The Global Burden of Disease (WHO, 2010) estimates that intravenous drug users (IDU) account for 10% of AIDS cases in some high incidence countries and that the largest individual cause of death for illicit drug users was AIDS (Degenhardt and Day, 2004). The rates of infection vary according to country. Aceijas et al. (2004) report HIV prevalence in IDU as high as 20% at sites in 25 countries and territories studied including: Estonia, Kazakhstan, Russia, Ukraine, Italy, Serbia and Montenegro, Spain, Libya, India, Malaysia, Myanmar, Nepal, Thailand, China, Argentina, Brazil, Uruguay, Puerto Rico, USA, and Canada; but only 1–3% in Australia, and with some of the greatest increases in Eastern Europe and Central Asia who also have often rudimentary palliative and other health services.

HIV is still a major cause of death in IDU and is affected by what is injected. This demographic changes as new injecting populations emerge in Eastern Europe and South-east Asia. Cocaine, amphetamine, and 'speedball' (cocaine and heroin) use has the highest prevalence of HIV acquisition (Doherty et al., 2000). European data shows that female IDU have higher death rates than males (Bargagli et al., 2001) but that taking Highly Active Anti-retroviral Therapy (HAART) reduces mortality (Gayet-Ageron et al., 2004). This presupposes that the IDU is able to access and adhere to the medication regime. These drugs are of course neither free nor readily available in many countries. More worryingly recent data shows that IDU concurrent infection of HIV and hepatitis C viral infection is running at 90 to 95% (Poynard, 2004). It should also be recognized that IDU will often mix drugs that will interact with HAART medication such as ritonavir and methamphetamine (Urbina and Jones, 2004), leading to vastly increased levels of methamphetamine and death in some cases.

Hepatitis C affects approximately 170 million people world-wide and up to 11% of chronic carriers will develop liver cirrhosis within 20 years (Law, 1999). Up to 90% of certain populations in HIV groups in Western Europe are hepatitis C positive (Limburg, 2004). In the USA in New York an 8-year follow-up study of IDU showed 9% death rate from cirrhosis (Friedman et al., 1996), and in Stockholm a similar group had 4% death rate over an 8-year period from cirrhosis (Galli and Musicco, 1994). Studies have also shown higher rates in women probably because of greater rates of needle sharing (Budd et al., 2002).

From this data we know that IDU patients have a greater risk of concomitant endocarditis—both bacterial and fungal (Karch, 2002)—and have a greater rate of Staphylococcus Aureus over Streptococcal infections (Carrel et al., 1993). These are patients who are often poor at accessing health care and are unlikely to be on viral treatment or known to liver units.

Data from different countries show remarkably different rates of death

In Italy 1.5% died from septic shock, 0.2% from tetanus, and 0.2% from endocarditis (Galli and Musicco, 1994), whereas in London 2.4% died from endocarditis (Oppenheimer et al., 1994). The reason for the difference is not clear. It is only a matter of time before this group present with all of the stigmata of liver failure and its inherent palliative care needs.

The evidence shows that this group has a marked disease burden but it is not just the disease itself that can cause difficulty in accessing services such as palliative care. IDU will often be homeless and be shelter dwellers. There is little in the way of evidence to show what their palliative needs might be. Roy et al. (2004) studied 1,013 street youths between the ages of 14 and 25 in a North American setting. Over a 5-year period 26 of this group died. This represented a standardized mortality ratio of 11.4. The most common causes of death were suicide and overdose. This is compared with a similar study done by Hwang (2000) taking men aged 18 and over (n = 8933) where the mortality rate ratio of shelter dwellers was 8.3 for the 18- to 24-year-old group. This showed that mortality rates were substantially higher than those of the poorest in the population, and the highest rate ratios were seen in the younger ages. Clearly this is a group with a much higher death rate than their 'homed' contemporaries.

The concern is that as this population ages so the risk of chronic illness such as Hepatitis and age related illnesses will surface. North American studies have compared age of death in homeless people across Atlanta, San Francisco, and Seattle. They found the average age of this population at death to be 44, 41, and 47 respectively. This compares with the national average in the States of 76.5 years (Song et al., 2007, 2010).

These data do not, however, relate directly to palliative care. There is little evidence base for the palliative care needs of substance misusers. A recent study examined a pilot project based in Ottawa that had set up a palliative care service within a hostel. The authors retrospectively assessed 28 deaths (Podymow et al., 2006). Interestingly the average age of death was 49 and average length of stay 120 days. This is significantly longer than in traditional hospice models and presumably reflects the difficulty in accessing ongoing services for this population. In this study and many others homelessness can be used as a surrogate marker for studying substance misuser populations (see Chapter 15 by Jones in this volume). All studies have described diseases that would normally be amenable to treatment or certainly seen as appropriate for palliation. However, these patients often find themselves in situations that are not amenable to care, let alone palliative care. Co-existing diagnoses of substance misuse and mental health problems lead to this group often being found dead in the street, living in squats or being taken into emergency departments at the very end of their lives. If drug related deaths in hospital are studied, it is found that there is little difference between drug and non drug users, with death rates being 21% and 20% respectively (International Centre for Drug Policy, 2009). In an age when 'Preferred Place of Care', 'choice', and home death are touted as the gold standard for end of life care, we seem to be failing this group, always supposing that they have somewhere to call home.

The project described by Podymow et al. (2006) exploring shelter-based palliative care for the homeless terminally ill was different in that it allowed users to continue to drink alcohol and take street drugs. This might have allowed greater access to its programme for users referred from shelters. The study had 89% male deaths and 89% were caucasian. This does not reflect other North American shelter populations but might have been a bias due to acceptance of 'difficult' patients. The diagnostic groupings also reflect those reported across the literature with 43% patients having alcoholic cirrhosis as the main cause of death. Hepatitis B and C accounted for 39.3% and 64.3% respectively; 43% were diagnosed as depressed and 39% had a diagnosis of schizophrenia.

Patients' use of substance

Table 18.1 shows the different drugs used by clients in the study. What is interesting is that the levels of 'no addiction' are so low and also that morphine is the only strong opioid of misuse. In North America in general the use of diamorphine is low compared to the UK, whereas the use of oxycodone is relatively high, but not described in this study. If we assume that the majority of the patients dying in the programme had a substance misuse history, we can learn a little of the symptomatology of this population.

Symptoms

The symptom burden is very similar to the non-using population and is reassuring in that it shows symptoms that are commonly dealt with in more mainstream palliative settings. See Table 18.2.

Drugs used

The same can be said for the medication used to control symptoms. There are really very few differences in the opioids used. See Table 18.3. These data show that this group has very similar symptomatology to the non-substance misuse group described

Table 18.1 Drugs used by clients in the study

Addiction	n	%
Tobacco	27	96
Alcohol	14	50
IV Drug	6	21
Any street drugs	13	46
More than one street drug	6	21
Benzodiazepines	2	7
Cocaine	5	18
Demerol	1	4
Marijuana	7	25
Morphine	4	14
No addiction	5	18

Reproduced with permission from Podymow et al., 2006.

by Twycross et al. in their book, *Symptom Management in Advanced Cancer* (2009). What is also interesting is that only 57.1% required a palliative care consultation. It might have been anticipated that the complexity of the medical problems would lead to difficult symptoms such as pain. The authors report that only one patient was poorly pain controlled. The 'home' death rate (i.e. within the hostel palliative care setting) is also remarkable in this population, where chaotic lives often work against the effective delivery of successful end of life care.

This study also managed to cost the savings the pilot achieved. This was carried out by looking at the actual costs and using an expert panel to cost like for like hospital admission values. For the Hospice programme the average cost was C$15,000 +/− 17,600. This compared with a comparative hospital cost of $64,600 +/− 76,800, p <0.001. The main saving was in the bed night cost of Hospital, $684, versus Hospice programme of $125. This clearly has considerable significance in health economies where financial accountability and governance are increasingly important.

Table 18.2 The symptom burden

Patient Care	n = 28	%
Main Symptoms		
Pain	25	89.2
Nausea	19	67.9
Confusion/stupor/coma	17	60.7
Shortness of breath	14	50
Headache	5	17.9

Reproduced with permission from Podymow et al., 2006.

Table 18.3 Medication used to control symptoms

Drug	n	Percentage needing palliative care
PRN morphine/codeine	16	57.1
Fentanyl patch	13	46.4
Regular morphine	7	25
Morphine infusion	4	14.3
Methadone	1	3.6
Palliative Care consultation	12	57.1
Number of medicines range	2–37	
Care Needs		
Incontinent urine	27	96.4
Washing	27	96.4
Transfer	26	92.9
Diabetic/low salt/nutrition	23	82.1
Incontinent bowel	22	78.6
Feeding assistance	21	75
Dressing	17	60.7
Place of death		
Hospice	23	82
Hospital	5	18

Reproduced with permission from Podymow et al., 2006.

Song et al. (2010) also showed that trying to undertake advance care planning with homeless people is difficult and there is little in the way of evidence to show that it translates into homeless and drug users dying where they want to.

How to prescribe for this population

- Know your patient. It is vitally important to screen for substance misuse. This will mean asking in a sensitive way about the possibility of prescribed medicine misuse, 'recreational' drug use and alcohol use. This should then be recorded so that all prescribers are aware of this as a potential problem. The patient might not be the user, and knowing who they spend time with is equally important. A young man with HIV needing opioids for his lymphoma might be passing these to his IDU father.

- Record and assess pain and other symptoms accurately, using well-validated tools. Consistency between professionals will help all involved and reduce the risk of one being played off against the other. Reassess frequently and document what has worked and what has not. Continued opioid prescribing for clearly documented non-opioid sensitive pain is not unheard of.

- Agree a single prescriber and disseminate this information.
- Agree amounts to be prescribed and an expectation as to how long this supply should last for.
- Be honest. Frank and open discussions between prescriber and patient about what is expected from both sides sets the ground rules. It is important to discuss what will happen if these rules are broken. Consider a written 'contract' that spells out the above.
- Be clear that you might need to request a urine specimen.
- Be prepared to stop prescribing. If this occurs you still have a duty of care which means a responsibility to find a different prescriber. In these circumstances you also have the right to pass on the details about the patient's substance misuse and the circumstances that have led to you ceasing prescribing.
- Use only long-acting opioids wherever possible.
- Limit the use of short-acting opioids to avoid tolerance.

Tips for prescribing in the palliative care setting

- Maximize non-opioid analgesia.
- Use non-drug treatments, e.g. acupuncture, massage.
- Pill count.
- Liaise with local substance misuse team and set goals that are realistic for the patient and agree them between you both.
- Have frequent team meetings for goal readjustment as necessary and agree multi-disciplinary membership.
- Treat pain properly. Large doses might be needed.
- Uncertain prescribers may withhold medication, leading to aberrant behaviour in patients.
- Withholding appropriate doses can lead to withdrawal and pseudo-addictive behaviour.
- Familiarize yourself with the terminology adopted by users both for the drugs and the practices associated with them.

What are the settings for delivering palliative care to this patient group?

We know that this population is often homeless and this has been explored elsewhere in this book. However the palliative patient will be in both hospital and hospice settings as well as at home. Many IDU will also be accessing care through drug and alcohol services and prison and mental health services. Little is known about these populations but recent surveys have shed some light on the extent of the problem (Ellison, 2008).

A London study by Davies (2010) reported that between 1986 and 2005, 25 inmates died in London prisons and 28% of these deaths were in hospices. Clearly more work has to be done to study substance misuse in dying populations in different settings.

Resources

◆ Guidance on prescribing for substance misusers: British Pain Society, *Chronic Pain Guidance*, August 2006.

◆ Palliative Care Formulary and Bulletin Board for clinical queries: www.palliative-drugs.com.

◆ The National Treatment agency for Substance Misuse, an English resource for professionals, carers, and clients: www.nta.nhs.uk/ndtms.aspx.

References

Aceijas, C., Stimson, G., Hickman, M., and Rhodes, T. (2004). Global overview of injecting drug use and HIV infection among injecting drug users. *AIDS*, **18**: 2295–2303.

Bargagli, A. M., Sperati, A., Davoli, F., Forastiere, F., and Perucci, C. A. (2001). Mortality among problem drug users in Rome: An 18 year follow up study, 1980–1997. *Addiction*, **96**: 1455–63.

Budd, J., Copeland, L., Elton, R. and Robertson, J. R. (2002). Hepatitis C infection in a cohort of injecting drug users: Past and present risk factors and the implications for educational and clinical management. *European Journal of General Practice*, **8**: 95–100.

Carrel, T., Schaffner, A., Vogt, P., Laske, A., Niederhauser, U., Scheider, J. et al. (1993). Endocarditis in intravenous drug addicts and HIV infected patients: Possibilities and limitations of surgical treatment. *Journal of Heart Valve Disease*, **2**: 140–7.

Davies, E. A., Seghal, A., Linklater, K., Heaps, K., Moran, C., Walford, C., et al. (2010). Cancer in the London Prison Population. *Journal of Public Health*, **32**(4): 526–31.

Degenhardt, L. and Day, C. (eds) (2004). *The Course and Consequences of the Heroin Shortage in New South Wales*. NDLERF Monograph No. 4. Adelaide: Australasian Centre for Policing Research.

Doherty, M. C., Garfein, R. S., Monterroso, E., Brown, D., and Vlahov, D. (2000). Correlates of HIV infection amongst young adult short term injection drug users. *AIDS*, **14**: 717–26.

Edwards, G. and Gross, M. M. (1976). Alcohol dependence: Provisional description of a clinical syndrome. *British Medical Journal*, **1**: 1058–61.

Ellison, N. (2008). *Mental Health and Palliative Care–A Literature Review*. London: Mental Health Foundation.

Friedman, L. N., Williams, M. T., Singh, T. P., and Friedman, T. R. (1996). Tuberculosis, AIDS, and death among substance abusers on welfare in New York City. *New England Journal of Medicine*, **334**: 828–33.

Galli, M. and Musicco, M. (1994). Mortality of intravenous drug users living in Milan, Italy: Role of HIV-1 infection. *AIDS*, **8**: 1457–63.

Gayet-Ageron, A., Baratin, D., Marceillac, E., and Allard, R. (2004). The AIDS epidemic in Lyon: Patient characteristics and defining illnesses between 1985 and 2000. *HIV Med*, **5**(3): 163–70.

Gough, E., Kemph, M., Graham, L., Manzanero, M., and Hook, E. (2010). HIV and hepatitis B and C incidence rates in us correctional populations and high risk groups: A systematic review and meta-analysis. *BMC Public Health*, **10**(1): 777.

Hoare, J. and Moon, D. (eds) (2010). *Drug Misuse Declared: Findings from the 2009/10 British Crime Survey*. Home Office Statistical Bulletin. London: Home Office.

Huang, C. N., Wu, D. J., and Chen, K. S. (1993). Acute myocardial infarction caused by transnasal inhalation of amphetamine. *Japanese Heart Journal*, **34**: 815–16.

Hwang, S. (2000). Mortality among men using homeless shelters in Toronto, Ontario. *JAMA*, **283**(16): 2152–7.

Hwang, S. (2001). Homelessness and health, *Canadian Medical Association Journal*, **164**: 229–33.

International Centre for Drug Policy. (2009). Drug related deaths in the UK, ANNUAL REPORT 2009. www.sgul.ac.uk.

Karch, S. B. (2002). *Karch's Pathology of Drug Abuse*, 3rd edn. Boca Raton, FL: CRC Press.

Law, M. (1999). Modelling the hepatitis C virus epidemic in Australia. Hepatitis C Virus Projections Working Group. *Journal of Gastroenterology and Hepatology*, **14**(11): 1100–7.

Limburg, W. (2004). Natural history, treatment and prevention of hepatitis C in injecting drug users: An overview. In J. Jager, W. Limburg, M. Kretzscmar, M. Postma, and L. Weissing (eds), *Hepatitis C and Injecting Drug Use: Impact, Costs and Policy Potions*. EMCDDA Monograph 7, pp 21–38. Luxembourg: Office for Official Publications of the European Communities.

Mulchandani, R., Hand, T., and Panesar, L. K. (2010). *Seizures of Drugs in England and Wales, 2009/10*. Home Office Statistical Bulletin. London: Home Office.

National Drug and Treatment Monitoring System Agency. (2010). *Statistics for drug Treatment Activity in England 2009–10*. University of Manchester, www.ndtms.net.

Oppenheimer, E., Tobutt, C., Taylor, C., and Andrew, T. (1994). Death and survival in a cohort of heroin addicts from London clinics: A 22-year follow up. *Addiction*, **89**: 1299–1308.

Podymow, T., Turnbull, J., and Coyle, D. (2006). Shelter-based palliative care for the homeless terminally ill. *Palliative Medicine*, **20**(2): 81–6.

Poynard, T. (2004). Recent developments in hepatitis C diagnostics and treatment. In J. Jager, W. Limburg, M. Kretzscmar, M. Postma, and L. Weissing (eds), *Hepatitis C and Injecting Drug Use: Impact, Costs and Policy Options*. EMCDDA Monograph 7, pp. 41–76. Luxembourg: Office for Official Publications of the European Communities.

Roy, A. (2001). Characteristics of cocaine dependent patients who attempt suicide. *American Journal of Psychiatry*, **158**: 1215–19.

Roy, E., Haley, N., Leclerc, P., Sochanski, B., Boudreau, J., Boivin, J.-F. (2004). Mortality in a cohort of street youth in Montreal. *JAMA*, **292**(5): 569–74.

Song, J., Bartels, D. M., Ratner, E. R., Alderton, L., Hudson, B., and Ahluwalia, J. S. (2007). Dying on the streets: Homeless persons' concerns and desires about end of life care. *Journal of General Internal Medicine*, **22**(4): 435–41.

Song, J., Ratner, E. R., Wall, M. M., Bartels, N., Ulvestad, D., Petroskas, M., et al. (2010). Effect of an end-of-life planning intervention on the completion of advance directives in homeless persons: A randomized trial. *Annals of Internal Medicine*, **153**: 76–84.

Twycross, R., Wilcock, A., and Toller, C. (2009). *Symptom Management in Advanced Cancer*, 4th edn. Abingdon, UK: Radcliffe Publishing.

Urbina, A. and Jones, K. (2004). Crystal methamphetamine, its analogues, and HIV infection: Medical and psychiatric aspects of a new epidemic. *Clinical Infectious Diseases*, **38**: 890–4.

UNAIDS. (2009). Report on the global HIV/AIDS epidemic 2009. Retrieved 2009 from www.unaids.org.

World Health Organization. (2000). *Management of Substance Abuse–The Global Burden*. www.who.int/substance_abuse/facts/global_burden.

World Health Organization. (2004). *Definition of Palliative Care*. http://www.who.int/cancer/palliative/definition/en/.

World Health Organization. (2010). *A Strategy to Halt and Reverse the HIV Epidemic among People Who Inject Drugs in Asia and the Pacific: 2010–2015*. Geneva: World Health Organization.

Chapter 19

Family carers and social difference

Kelli I. Stajduhar

Introduction

Family carers are individuals who provide unpaid care and/or support to a family member, friend, neighbour, or significant other who has a physical or mental disability, is chronically ill, or is frail. In many resource rich countries the de-institutionalization of health and social care and increasing emphasis on care in the home has resulted in family carers taking on a large portion of the care that was once provided by the health and social care system. In England there are an estimated 5 million carers (Health and Social Care Information Centre, 2010). In Canada, 1.5 to 2 million carers provide $25–26 billion worth of care annually (Hollander, Liu, et al., 2009). Coined the 'invisible welfare state', the unpaid contributions of family carers have been estimated to be five times the paid workforce in terms of full-time equivalents (Australian Institute of Health and Welfare, 2003). Clearly, family carers provide a substantial service to the health and social care system and to society at large. This is particularly true in resource poor countries where access to services is severely limited and where family members may be the only people available to provide care (Hunt, 2009).

The rising number of people facing old age makes it likely that serious chronic and life-limiting illness will be a dominant challenge for health care delivery in the next half-century. Family carers will continue to play a major role in the provision of support and care. In this chapter I briefly summarize what is known about family carers to lay the foundation to engage in discussions of difference. Specifically, I will discuss 'social differences' that receive relatively little attention in the literature in relation to family care work: cultural and religious difference, and social class difference. I will use examples to illustrate how these differences can challenge that which we have learned about carers and will suggest supportive interventions that take into account such difference.

Family care work at the end of life

While men are increasingly engaged in caregiving functions, women provide the large majority of care to chronically ill and dying people (Armstrong, Amaratunga, et al., 2002). Carers cross the age span, but most carers are middle-aged (National Alliance for Caregiving, 2004), are employed in addition to their unpaid family care work (Ferrario, Cardillo, et al., 2004) or stop working temporarily or reduce their paid work in order to provide care (Hudson, 2004). Most research on family carers at the end of life relates to carers of people with cancer. There is less known about those who provide care to people with other serious life-limiting illnesses (Stajduhar, Funk, et al., 2010).

Family care work offers considerable rewards as the process of giving care can facilitate closure after the death and help carers find meaning in their experiences (Salmon, Kwak, et al., 2005). Moderate to high levels of emotional and psychological difficulty, financial strain, activity disruptions, and negative physical health outcomes are also common (Stajduhar, Funk, et al., 2010). The caregiving experience is uncertain because of the unpredictability of the trajectory (Farber, Egnew, et al., 2003); there is a disruption to 'normal life' (Stajduhar and Davies, 2005) and experiences of helplessness, vulnerability, and isolation are common (Milberg, Strang, et al., 2005). Getting support is often hampered because many family carers do not identify themselves as legitimate recipients of help. Long hours of care provision are accompanied by fatigue and sleep deprivation. Family carers may feel ill-prepared for caregiving roles and uncertain about their abilities (Wennman-Larsen and Tishelman, 2002); some feel pressured to provide such care yet feel ambivalent about it (Stajduhar and Davies, 2005).

The challenges associated with family care work are primarily related to the work involved in the care of the dying which includes, but is not limited to: (a) conducing domestic chores and household tasks; (b) providing personal care and assisting the dying person with activities of daily living; (c) managing symptoms such as pain and constipation; (d) providing emotional and social support to the dying person; (e) being a spokesperson, advocate, and proxy decision-maker; and (f) coordinating all aspects of the dying person's care (Stajduhar and Cohen, 2009). The challenges that carers face are exacerbated in resource poor countries where poverty and illness are rampant and where palliative care services are scarce (Hunt, 2009).

Family care work and social difference

Regardless of age, gender, disease, geographic locale, and other variations of caregiving characteristics, there is some universality in the experience of family carers. There are also important social differences. Here I focus on cultural and religious difference and social class difference.

Cultural and religious difference

Our world is home to an increasingly diverse population. Whereas in the past, resource rich countries were populated by the dominant (white) culture, this is no longer the case (Kagawa-Singer and Blackhall, 2010). Many resource rich countries are now home to an increasingly large immigrant population who come with distinct values, beliefs, and cultural and religious practices that often differ from those in resource rich nations. These differences have implications for how we conceptualize family care work. For instance, many members of recent immigrant communities are embedded in traditional cultural and religious communities (e.g. Muslim, Hindu, Sikh, Buddhist, and traditional Chinese) in which the autonomous 'I-self' (Coward and Ratanakul, 1999), that is central to the way families and individual autonomy are understood in the West, is held to be of much less significance than the socially interconnected 'we-self'.

Whereas the dominant model at work in many North American social settings presupposes that the locus of identity and decision making is the individual, in we-self cultures, major end of life decisions, such as who should provide end of life care, are understood to be the rightful topics of concern for a broad network of family and friends. Conflicts between the dominant 'I-self' culture and that characterized as the 'we-self' may arise where tensions can emerge between those of the first generation who may be closely tied to traditional ethnic and religious values and those of the second and third generations who may have a more liberal and individualistic approach to their personal, cultural, and religious identities. For example, it is not at all uncommon to have dying (relative) newcomer Canadians cared for in the home by second or third generation children and grandchildren who may not espouse the same traditional religious and cultural values and practices. Such caregiving contexts can engender tremendous stress and resentment in the lives of the carers when they are asked, or in fact expected, to set aside many of the individualistic values they have embraced for decades in order to respect traditional patriarchal, religious and ethnic values and practices.

Relatedly, while language and communication barriers are often cited as reasons why carers from ethnic minority groups may not access services at the end of life (Kagawa-Singer and Blackhall, 2010), issues of filial responsibility should also be considered. Filial piety, or the expectation that children will care for their parents without question, is an important concept, particularly in Asian cultures. Among Chinese families, for example, caregiving is an essential element of filial piety and acceptance of hospice care by carers can be considered dishonourable to the parents as it sends a message to their larger community that the family is unable to provide adequate care. As Kagawa-Singer and Blackhall (2010) maintain, how well carers fulfil their filial obligations is 'open to community scrutiny and judgement and would reflect poorly on the parenting abilities of the parents and on the extended family if the children do not fulfil their obligations' (p. 340). In this instance, interventions commonly offered to carers such as respite care, visiting nurses, or help with practical aspects of caregiving in the home, may not be welcome suggestions and in fact may be viewed as insulting.

Conflicts may also emerge between family carers and professional care providers when traditional cultural and religious ways are not understood by providers. In palliative care, this is often seen in relation to truth-telling. For example, in some Chinese traditions, families will not discuss death and dying with the patient for fear of invoking bad luck (Yick and Gupta, 2002) and sometimes, providers are asked by the carer to not tell the ill person of their impending death. These approaches are in contrast to a westernized approach that supports the belief that the dying be informed of their impending death. In such conflicts, one may witness differences between what we might call religious culture, which may include distinctive rituals, languages, texts, assumptions, and hierarchies, and what is arguably a professional/expert culture, offering their understanding of cultural and religious care.

Social class differences

Although socio-demographic and economic attributes do not emerge as potent independent influences on various caregiving outcomes, it would be erroneous to assume that the impact of caregiving is not dependent upon the carer's characteristics or locations in the social system. Family care work is embedded within the context of a carer's life and his or her social standing. Even in a country like Canada with well-established palliative care programmes, only 16 to 30 per cent of Canadians who die, and their carers, have access to or receive palliative care services, and even fewer carers receive grief and bereavement care (Canadian Institutes of Health Information, 2007). There are many reasons for this and some research suggests that social class differences play a role. For example, people with lower levels of education, unskilled employment, and in lower social classes are less likely to access formal health services, relying instead on informal networks (Pinquart and Sorensen, 2005). Low-income carers have increased needs for support and education compared to those who can afford to pay for services beyond those provided by the state and they experience greater carer distress than do carers in higher income brackets (Williams, Forbes, et al., 2003). A growing body of research indicates that ethnic minorities lack access to treatment for symptoms such as pain (Cleeland, Goin, et al., 1997) and barriers to health and social care that the poor and disenfranchised have traditionally encountered may affect the patient and carer's receptivity to palliative care. At the same time, family carers who do not access formal services and have minimal support tend to experience more stress and burden than those with more support (Grbich, Parker, et al., 2001; Knight, Devereux, et al., 1997).

In addition to these differences, overlooked populations such as those who are homeless and dying on the streets conjure up different definitions of family carers. Since many homeless persons are reluctant to contact families towards the end of life and avoid hospitalization, those taking on the caregiving role may be other homeless people who have mental health and/or addictions issues, personnel working in shelters or transition houses, or street outreach workers, many of whom who are unprepared for providing care at the end of life and who may be overwhelmed by witnessing multiple 'bad deaths' (Podymow, Turnbull, et al., 2006; Stajduhar, Poffenroth, et al., 2004). There is a paucity of literature available to direct us to how to best support these carers who themselves can feel stigmatized and marginalized because of the populations of people that they care for.

Finally, some of the most noticeable differences among the experience of carers are between those caring in resource rich and resource poor countries. Kellehear (2009) points out that for regions such as Africa, the provision of end of life care is heavily dependent on family carers because access to health services is severely limited. Diseases such as HIV/AIDS are highly stigmatized and carers may themselves experience shame, stigma and social isolation and rejection by association, leaving families with even fewer social and material supports. Widespread poverty, civil unrest, political uncertainty, and access to the basic necessities of life such as clean drinking water all provide a challenging backdrop upon which end of life care is provided. In resource rich countries with established palliative care services, carers tend to be of a higher social class, have more economic resources and access to specialized services. In resource poor countries, carers tend to be of a lower social class, live in rural areas, have few economic resources and limited or no access to specialized services (Hunt, 2009). While family carers in resource rich settings experience many burdens associated with care work, this is even more pronounced in resource poor countries. Children affected by HIV/AIDS take on a major portion of family care work, oftentimes needing to stop schooling to take on family domestic chores once reserved for adults or to provide care to sick and dying parents and relatives (Hunt, 2009).

Social difference and supportive interventions for carers

Although family carers provide the vast majority of care at the end of life, they typically receive little preparation, information or support to undertake this vital role. Several carer interventions have been implemented to reduce the negative impacts of caregiving and enhance the positive aspects. Northhouse and colleagues (2010) conducted a meta-analysis of 29 randomized trials of interventions (psycho-educational, skills training, and therapeutic counselling) with family carers of cancer patients and found that even though effects were small to moderate in size, the interventions showed promise in achieving clinically significant outcomes such as reduced burden, enhanced capacity to cope, and improved quality of life. As the authors highlight, however, there are few interventions that study racial, cultural and socioeconomic diversity, with only two of the 29 studies tailored for a particular cultural or racial group. There is a need for future studies that focus on the inherent diversities in family care work and that will better inform the development of supportive interventions in this regard. As a starting point, providers can acknowledge that cultural and religious diversity is an important part of the fabric of palliative care, regardless of the country in which one resides. Understanding cultural and religious diversity is not, however, just about learning a set of beliefs or practices of an ethnic group or religious tradition. In making such categorizations we 'run the risk of stereotyping or believing we know what any one individual thinks or does because we assume we know what people of that group tend to think' (Kagawa-Singer and Blackhall, 2010: 331). Recognizing that there can be wide variation in beliefs and practices for individuals within particular groups will enhance the likelihood of individual needs being attended to.

Despite the challenges faced by carers in resource poor countries, Wright (2003) illustrates how countries such as Russia and Swaziland have developed imaginative models to provide better end of life care to the dying. Though much more is required to ensure access to palliative care services that will be supportive of carers worldwide, Hunt (2009) maintains that educating health professionals and the large voluntary sector as well as enhancing access to analgesics will help to improve the quality of dying and support for carers, particularly in rural and remote settings where access to specialized services in nonexistent. Additionally, as Kellehear (2009) argues, supporting community development initiatives is a necessity in resource poor countries where non-professional supports are sometimes the only supports available. While there are implications to adopting empowerment and health promoting principles within the context of family caregiving at the end of life (Stajduhar, Funk, et al., 2010), an approach that incorporates health promotion, community empowerment and development and partnerships with service organizations (if they are available) will be crucial to support carers in resource poor countries.

Conclusion

Family care work for dying individuals presents distinct challenges and is clearly associated with economic, social, cultural, gender, and religious forces. For the most part, the contributions of these carers are uncompensated and under-recognized despite considerable academic knowledge on the risk of negative social, financial, emotional, and physical impacts of providing care to dying individuals. Care demands can be particularly onerous towards the end of life, and emotional stresses particularly high as family members grieve successive losses, awareness of impending death; and an uncertain future. For family carers outside the 'mainstream', the challenges are exacerbated. Yet, the social history of dying indicates that families have always cared for each other (Kellehear, 2009). Perhaps we have something to learn from those family carers not in the 'mainstream'—those who are socially diverse. In doing so we may, in fact, become more creative with the ways in which we serve family carers at the end of life.

Resources

- International Palliative Care Family Carer Research Collaboration (IPCFRC). www.ipcfrc.unimelb.edu.au
- Payne, S., and her colleagues from the EAPC Task Force on Family Carers. (2010). White paper on improving support for family carers in palliative care. www.eapc-net.eu/Themes/Specificgroups/Familycarers/Taskforcepublications/tabid/732/Articleid/192/mid/1443/Default.aspx
- Hunt, J. (2009). Family carers in resource-poor countries. In P. Hudson and S. Payne (eds), *Family Carers in Palliative Care*. Oxford: Oxford University Press, 72–92.

References

Armstrong, P., Amaratunga, C., Bernier, J., Grant, K., Pederson, A., and Willson, K. (2002). *Exposing Privatization: Women and Health Care Reform in Canada*. Aurora: Garamond Press.

Australian Institute of Health & Welfare. (2003). *The Future Supply Of Informal Care 2003 to 2013: Alternative Scenarios: A Report Jointly Funded by the Australian Government Department of Health and Ageing and the Australian Institute of Health and Welfare*. Canberra: Australian Institute of Health and Welfare.

Canadian Institutes of Health Information. (2007). *Health Care Use at the End of Life in Western Canada*. Ottawa, ON: CIHI.

Cleeland, C. S., Goin, R., Baez, L., Loehrer, P., and Pandya, K. J. (1997). Pain and treatment of pain in minority patients with cancer: The Eastern Cooperative Oncology Group Minority Outpatient Pain Study. *Annals of Internal Medicine*, **127**: 813–16.

Coward, H., and Ratanakul, P. (eds). (1999). *A Cross-cultural Dialogue on Health Care Ethics*. Waterloo, ON: Wilfred Laurier University Press.

Farber, S. J., Egnew, T. R., Herman-Bertsch, J. L., Taylor, T. R. and Guldin, G. E. (2003). Issues in end-of-life care: Patient, caregiver, and clinician perceptions. *Journal of Palliative Medicine*, **6**(1): 19–31.

Ferrario, S. R., Cardillo, V., Vicario, F., Balzarini, E., and Zotti, A. M. (2004). Advanced cancer at home: Caregiving and bereavement. *Palliative Medicine*, **18**(2): 129–36.

Grbich, C., Parker, D., and Maddocks, I. (2001). The emotions and coping strategies of caregivers of family members with terminal cancer. *Journal of Palliative Care*, 17: 30–6.

Health and Social Care Information Centre. (2010). Survey of carers in households in England 2009/10. London: The Information Centre for Health and Social Care. Available at: www.ic.nhs.uk/webfiles/publications/Social%20Care/carersurvey0910/Survey_of_Carers_in_Households_2009_10_England_Provisional_Results_post_publication.pdf (accessed 1 Nov. 2010).

Hollander, M. J., Liu, G., and Chappell, N. L. (2009). Who cares about how much? The imputed economic contribution to the Canadian healthcare system of middle aged and older unpaid caregivers providing care to the elderly. *Healthcare Quarterly*, 12(2): 42–59.

Hudson, P. (2004). Positive aspects and challenges associated with caring for a dying relative at home. *International Journal of Palliative Nursing*, 10(2): 58–65.

Hunt, J. (2009). Family carers in resource-poor countries. In P. Hudson and S. Payne (eds), *Family Carers in Palliative Care*. Oxford: Oxford University Press, 72–92.

Kagawa-Singer, M., and Blackhall, L. J., (2010). Negotiating cross-cultural issues at the end of life—'You got to go where he lives'. In D. E. Meier, S. L. Isaacs, and R. G. Hughes (eds), *Palliative Care: Transforming the Care of Serious Illness*. Princeton, NJ: Jossey-Bass, 330–47.

Kellehear, A. (2009). Understanding social and cultural dimensions of family caregiving. In P. Hudson and S. Payne (eds), *Family Carers in Palliative Care*. Oxford: Oxford University Press, 21–36.

Knight, R. G., Devereux, R. C., and Godfrey, H. P. D. (1997). Psychosocial consequences of caring for a spouse with multiple sclerosis. *Journal of Clinical and Experimental Neuropsychology*, 19: 7–19.

Milberg, A., Strang, P., and Jackobsson, M. (2005). Next of kin's experience of powerlessness and helplessness in palliative home care. *Supportive Care in Cancer*, 12(2): 120–8.

National Alliance for Caregiving. (2004). *Caregiving in the US*. Washington, DC: AARP.

Northhouse, L. L., Katapodi, M. C., Song, L., Zhang, L., and Mood, D. W. (2010). Interventions with family caregivers of cancer patients: Meta-analysis of randomized trials. *CA: A Cancer Journal for Clinicians*, 60(5): 317–39.

Pinquart, M. and Sorensen, S. 2005. Ethnic differences in stressors, resources, and psychological outcomes of family caregiving: A meta-analysis. *The Gerontologist*, 45(1): 90–106.

Polymow, T., Turnbull, J., and Coyle, D. (2006). Shelter-based palliative care for the homeless terminally ill. *Palliative Medicine*, 20: 81–6.

Salmon, J. R., Kwak, J., Acquaviva, K. D., Brandt, K., and Egan, K. A. (2005). Transformative aspects of caregiving at life's end. *Journal of Pain and Symptom Management*, 29(2): 121–9.

Stajduhar, K. I., Poffenroth, L., Wong, E., Archibald, C. P., Sutherland, D., and Rekart, M. (2004). Missed opportunities: Injection drug use and HIV/AIDS in Victoria, Canada. *International Journal of Drug Policy*, 15: 171–81.

Stajduhar, K. and Cohen, R. (2009). Family caregiving in the home. In P. Hudson and S. Payne (eds), *Family Carers in Palliative Care*. Oxford: Oxford University Press, 149–68.

Stajduhar, K. I. and Davies, B. (2005). Variations in and factors influencing family members' decisions for palliative home care. *Palliative Medicine*, 19(1): 21–32.

Stajduhar, K. I., Funk, L., Jakobsson, E., and Öhlén, J. (2010). A critical analysis of health promotion and 'empowerment' in the context of palliative family caregiving. *Nursing Inquiry*, 17(3): 221–30.

Stajduhar, K. I., Funk, L., Toye, C., Aoun, S., Grande, G., and Todd, C. (2010). Part 1: Home-based family caregiving at the end of life: A comprehensive review of published quantitative research (1998–2008). *Palliative Medicine*, **26**(6): 573–93.

Wennman-Larsen, A. and Tishelman, C. (2002). Advanced home care for cancer patients at the end of life: A qualitative study of hopes and expectations of family caregivers. *Scandinavian Journal of Caring Sciences*, **16**(3): 240–7.

Williams, A., Forbes, D., Mitchell, J., Essar, M., and Corbett, B. (2003). The influence of income on the experience of informal caregiving: Policy implications. *Health Care for Women International*, **24**: 280–91.

Wright, M. (2003). *Models of Hospice and Palliative Care in Resource Poor Countries: Issues and Opportunities*. Lancaster, UK: Help the Hospices.

Yick, A. G. and Gupta, R. (2002). Chinese cultural dimensions of death, dying, and bereavement: Focus group findings. *Journal of Cultural Diversity*, **9**(2): 32–42.

Chapter 20

Sexual orientation

Katherine Cox

Introduction

In this chapter I consider sexual orientation as an issue of social difference in relation to death, dying, and bereavement. Some of the excluded groups explored in this book are clearly visible—'Outed' by their very physicality and/or context. Our sexual orientation, on the other hand, whilst key to self-understanding and social role, is a private, hidden aspect of ourselves that we may choose, or not, to share with others. Our sexual roles carry particular social meanings, and social expectations and norms may or may not validate experience. I explore the experience of lesbian, gay, bisexual, and transgender (LGBT) communities within palliative care to argue that these groups are disenfranchised within particular socio-cultural norms of what it means to experience end of life loss. I argue that a more open and flexible response is required from practitioners to allow people their unique narrative.

LGBT communities—the socio-historical and cultural context

Over the last thirty years a significant body of literature has emerged regarding LGBT communities; health within those communities; the social and political context of health need; and the services providing assistance to those communities. Same sex experience has undergone radically different constructions through history.

Lesbian, gay, bisexual, and transgender are convenient terms, or 'fictions' (Plummer, 1992; Weeks, 1995) requiring deconstruction or at least problematizing. Yet a pragmatic focus on quality of service provision is also required, and in order to do this effectively, the population requires definition.

When we ask 'Are LGBT clients disenfranchised within palliative care services?' we are asking a political and social question to be addressed at the level of policy and systems; an intrapersonal question about patients', families', and professionals' understandings of identity and the locus of the erotic within that identity; and we are asking a question about the interplay of those understandings within services.

Whichever focus is taken, it is striking to note that almost all the prevailing research demonstrates that LGBT communities have poorer mental and physical health than heterosexual groups; the incidence of suicide and self-harm is higher and drug and alcohol problems are more prevalent (King et al., 2003a,b, 2006). For gay and bisexual men in particular, these issues have been played out against the backdrop of HIV.

The historical context

Some of the historical changes in relation to LGBT experiences in the UK have been significant and tumultuous but not without oppressive backlash. In 1967 the Sexual Offences Act partially decriminalized sex between men over 21. In 1969 the Stonewall Riot began in New York, echoed in 1970 by the formation of the UK-based Gay Liberation Front. Yet in 1988 section 28 of the Local Government Act came into force, preventing the 'promotion' of homosexual orientation by local authorities. The age of consent for sex between two men was reduced from 21 to 18 in 1994 and to 16 in 2001 and male rape was made a criminal offence. In 2003 section 28 was repealed and in the same year Employment Equality (Sexual Orientation) Regulations made it illegal to discriminate against LGB people in the workplace. In 2004 the Civil Partnerships Act was passed.

It is important to acknowledge how recent these changes have been. A 53-year-old gay man will have been 10 years old, and quite possibly aware of his sexual orientation, when sex between men was still illegal. Legislative change is vital but it is a slower matter to change cultural understandings and values and whilst recent advances in sexual politics have been impressive, those within healthcare services have been slower. Changes in legislation and terminology do not necessarily reflect changed paradigms.

The political context

UK government white papers on mental health, 'The Health of the Nation' (DoH, 1992) and 'Saving lives: our healthier nation' (DoH, 1999) are silent on LGBT issues although mental health difficulties amongst LGBT communities are known to be very high (King et al., 2003, 2006). Similarly, the NICE Guidelines (DoH, 2004) do not mention sexual orientation. The extent of the health need within the LGBT community remains, despite the research evidence, unrecognized and unacknowledged at the level of policy and service provision. Interestingly, much more information has been produced for trans people (www.spectrumlondon.org.uk/DHBooklets.htm).

Patients and staff will enter a palliative care service with a particular experience and understanding of sexual orientation which is politically, historically, and culturally constructed. This will form judgements, values and expectations which may be more or less consciously held. LGBT patients will already have experienced generic health care provision and their expectations of palliative care services will be influenced by their healthcare history.

The international context

This chapter is written from a UK perspective but of course the picture is different across different countries and societies. The International Gay and Lesbian Human Rights Commission (www.iglhrc.org) and Amnesty International (www.amnestyusa.org/lgbt-human-rights/country-information/page.do?id=1106576) give information regarding the cultural, legal and political position for lesbian and gay people internationally.

Taking one example, anti-LGBT sentiment in the Caribbean is strongly influenced by Christian and Rastafari beliefs; popular cultural views expressed through media such as reggae and dancehall; and prevailing masculine norms. Article 79 of the

Jamaican Criminal Code punishes men who commit any act of 'gross indecency' with another male in public or private with up to two years imprisonment with or without hard labour (Amnesty International, 2010).

On the other side of the Atlantic Ocean, homosexuality is criminalized in both Nigeria and Uganda. Here, prevailing legislation (for example Chapter 42, section 214 of Nigeria's criminal code, penalizing same sex activity) is reinforced by Sharia penal codes.

In such contexts, LGBT individuals facing life-threatening illness are compelled to hide their sexual orientation, their partner, aspects of their lifestyle and culture.

The academic/research context

There is a significant lack of research concerning the specific experiences of lesbians and gay men in palliative care services. The body of literature on sexuality and health care from a heterosexual perspective (e.g. Field et al., 1997; Oliviere et al., 1998) is a welcome contribution to the field in that it acknowledges the importance of considering sex and sexuality in the provision of holistic care. This work does not, however, consider the particular experience of LGBT communities.

The much more significant body of literature on palliative care for gay men with HIV (e.g. Colburn and Malena, 1988; Sherr, 1995; Fisher et al., 1996; Kellerhouse, 1996) can in many ways translate to the experience of lesbians and gay men facing or affected by other life-threatening conditions but there is no literature which takes account of the differences. HIV is a specific social experience carrying a specific social weight. Lesbians and gay men with other life-threatening conditions will have a qualitatively different experience from those who are HIV positive. Much of what has been written about palliative care and HIV in any case is out of date given the changes brought about by anti-retroviral therapy. The literature cited above dates from a period when most gay men with AIDS had a very short prognosis compared to the current context of prolonged prognosis and better health.

Exclusion and invisibility

Multiple exclusion

To be ill, dying, or bereaved is in itself a socially excluding experience, both practically and psychologically. LGBT clients within palliative care thus face multiple layers of exclusion and may feel excluded from their own communities.

Jon was a gay man and night club owner. When he became ill with prostate cancer he lost his business and the strong community links it gave him. When Jon died, his partner Gary could no longer participate in the nightclub scene and became isolated and withdrawn. The hospice bereavement worker extended the number of sessions and together they looked at alternative ways Gary could socialize. In time, Gary retrained as a care worker and joined a gay men's hiking club.

Unrecognized loss

LGBT clients using bereavement care services may experience 'disenfranchised loss' (Doka, 1989). The very nature of this type of grief exacerbates the pain of bereavement, but the usual sources of support may not be available or helpful. Grief may be disenfranchised because the relationship is not recognized and therefore the loss is not recognized (see also Chapter 22 by Keegan in this volume).

Social norms specify who can grieve, how much, for how long, and in what way. Those who have lost a same sex partner are not necessarily accorded the same rights and privileges in the expression of grief as heterosexual partners. In addition, there is a connection between being given permission and giving oneself permission to grieve. Bereaved LGBT clients may themselves struggle to recognize the full extent of their loss when they receive no validation from others. People may be unable to say at work or to friends/family that their same sex partner has died. When a heterosexual spouse dies, the surviving partner has a recognized social role of widow/er which carries social status and legal and social rights; bereaved spouses may have time off work, apply for benefits, they are excused certain social responsibilities and permitted a wider range of emotional expression. All of these may be denied a same sex partner.

Marie is bisexual. She is married to John and in addition has had an enduring relationship with Joyce for 21 years. When Joyce dies Marie's friends and work colleagues assume she has simply lost a close friend. Marie is unable to talk to anyone about her devastating sense of grief. The Macmillan nurse who cared for Joyce visits Marie and together they light a candle and share memories. She is also able to explain to Marie the details of Joyce's last hours as Marie was unable to share them with her.

Assumptions of heterosexuality

An LGBT client not only has to manage actual and feared homophobic prejudice but in addition a far more pervasive experience of heterosexism—the assumption that they are heterosexual. An assumption of heterosexuality in effect renders a key aspect of that person's identity as invisible and potentially unsayable.

Fiona is admitted to the hospice with advanced metastatic breast cancer. She is accompanied by her partner Sarah. The doctor clerking her in asks about next of kin and, turning to Fiona says, 'You're her daughter I presume?' A lesbian nurse, who is not open about her sexuality at work, overhears the remark. Later she quietly takes the doctor aside to discuss the implications of his assumption and speaks to the hospice manager about organizing some team-wide LGBT awareness training.

Fear of stigma/actual stigma

Whilst services may be making efforts to improve attitudes to LGBT users, cultural change is slow to effect and the fear of discrimination may prevent LGBT individuals from using services freely. Many LGBT individuals choose not to disclose their sexual orientation to their service provider (Bybee and Roeder, 1990, in Dean et al., 2000; see also Fitzpatrick et al., 1994) and difficulty in communicating with providers is associated with delay in seeking health care (Harrison, 1996, White and Dull, 1998, in Dean et al., 2000). King et al. (2003) identify in their study some exceptionally discriminatory attitudes held by health care providers. They are careful to argue that this is increasingly rare but the fact that it is possible perpetuates anxiety and fear amongst

LGBT individuals. They also noted that many of the participants had such low expectations, that they reported experiences as positive which another person would not; there was simply not an expectation of equality.

Relationships with others, relationship with self

Partners: relationships and relationship conflict

It can be harder to acknowledge difficulties within a relationship when the couple feel they have to justify themselves. LGBT clients may struggle to ask for and receive support in circumstances which can place a great strain on a relationship.

Stella and Joan have lived together for 2 years. Joan's family strongly disapprove. Stella was diagnosed with cancer soon after they met and the relationship has been under a great deal of strain with her deteriorating health. The couple have been arguing but Joan feels she cannot say or do anything because then she would have proved her family right. The homecare team arrange for Stella and Joan to speak to a counsellor both together and separately.

Families

Whilst LGBT communities are in no way monolithic, for many these communities are their 'family' of choice. In many cases there is a good relationship between an LGBT partner and birth family and they can provide an important support for each other. In other cases the relationship is a source of stress and conflict. People may be forced at the point of illness to tell their families they are LGBT, or may choose never to disclose their sexual orientation which can cause stress and confusion after death.

Many LGBT people distance themselves both geographically and emotionally from their parents and bridging the gap can be challenging for all parties. Sometimes only certain family members know and family secrets can cause even more distress. Parents may feel anger at their child's sexuality especially if they feel it has contributed to their child's death in the case of HIV, and if they learn about both at the same time, the two are more likely to be conflated. As mourners they may also be stigmatized; parents who may be homophobic may themselves become the target of homophobic prejudice. Their anger can then easily be projected on the surviving partner.

Relationships with other patients

Hospices and nursing homes are communities and patients/loved ones create relationships not only with staff but with each other which may be supportive or damaging/unhelpful.

Rituals and Faith

People from LGBT communities may find themselves on the fringe or outside their particular religious communities and may not be able to draw on the very source of support they need. Funerals are significant spaces within which the deceased person's sexuality and bereaved partner/friends can be publicly validated. Acknowledging all aspects of the person's life and all their relationships can, however, present a significant challenge. Families may forbid the partner from attending the service, and refuse to disclose the nature of the death to relatives if it was the result of HIV.

Barry is Catholic. He lived with his 'friend', Marshall, for 50 years before Marshall's death from prostate cancer. Barry cannot pray, nor talk to his priest about his loss because he believes that to be gay is a sin. The bereavement counsellor arranges for him to meet with the priest attached to the hospice. A Mass is said for Marshall and they plant a tree in his memory.

Bereavement—loss of partner, loss of identity

Loss of a partner can often precipitate a sense of lost identity and for LGBT clients this can be a complex experience of loss of sexual identity. If someone has defined themselves as LGBT largely through their relationship, the loss of that relationship renders that part of themselves once again invisible. Some clients may feel 'de-sexualized', whilst others may seek sexual encounters in order once again to feel that part of themselves.

Dying—different and changing relationship with sex and sexuality

The changes associated with illness and bereavement can have a significant impact on a person's social, political and sexual identity. Changes in the physical self can threaten a person's sense of belonging in the gay community with its emphasis on youth, beauty and health. Loss of sexual activity/function through illness or bereavement can undermine the individual's sexual identity.

Different contexts, different challenges

Many people choose to die at home which involves accepting a large number of professionals in one's personal space, all of whom will notice their surroundings and draw particular conclusions and judgements. For an LGBT patient, this may lead to a dilemma between hiding items associated with one's sexual orientation or outing oneself to every visiting professional with associated further loss of privacy. This dilemma between privacy and disclosure also faces those in hospital and nursing home care.

Minorities within minorities

Bisexual communities

For bisexual communities the research is scant, but it is clear that bisexual men and women are vulnerable to rejection both from heterosexual and from gay and lesbian groupings (Savin-Williams and Cohen, 1996) and it is more difficult for those who identify as bisexual to find spaces, services and communities.

In a palliative care context, someone's bisexuality may be 'hidden' behind a public exterior of heterosexuality and clients may have other partners, communities and lives which are less publicly lived. On the other hand, the patient may be open about their bisexual identity but this may be problematic for others around them.

Lesbian women

Results of several studies (Bradford and Ryan, 1988; Bradford et al., 1994) found that lesbians are reluctant to seek healthcare and/or have had negative experiences with healthcare providers. This may mean that a lesbian may present far later and perhaps be more anxious about the quality of the treatment she will receive; whether her definition of her family will be respected and whether appropriate social and psychological support will be available for her and significant others. The voice of lesbians can be silenced or simply 'tagged on' to gay men's issues when in fact lesbian experience will be qualitatively different both from heterosexual women and gay men. Lesbian women may well have children to consider and may be afraid that disclosure will jeopardize wishes for future child care arrangements. Health care professionals may be more aware of the needs of gay men as a result of HIV but may demonstrate a marked lack of awareness of the needs of lesbian patients and partners.

Trans communities

Although the umbrella term LGBT makes pragmatic sense, there are compelling arguments to treat transgendered people as distinct from LGB communities: gender identity is clearly distinct from sexual identity (Dean et al., 2000) and to conflate the two risks ignoring the particular experiences of this group which is itself heterogeneous, comprising intersex individuals, androgynes, transvestites, and a whole range of others. Transgendered people can experience significant barriers to health care services (ibid.) due to service providers' views that transgender experience is pathological, similarly they can experience trans-phobia within LGB services and communities. In addition, service providers are often ignorant about trans issues so an educative burden is placed on the client. Transgender individuals are more likely to experience shame, low self-esteem, isolation, loneliness, anxiety, and depression than heterosexual controls (Prieur, 1990, in Dean et al., 2000) but at levels comparable to groups who have experienced major life changes, relationship difficulties, chronic medical conditions, or significant discrimination. Rates of substance misuse and suicide are also high (ibid.). Studies also evidence high levels of distress experienced by the partners of transgendered people (Cole, 1999, Doctor and Prince, 1997, in Dean et al., 2000).

In a palliative care context transgendered people risk being misunderstood, having all aspects of their well-being filtered through their transgendered gender identity and being exoticized and/or criticized.

Practical measures

There are concrete ways in which we can assist LGBT clients facing life-threatening conditions in promoting and securing their rights and wishes within a social context of exclusion.

Wills

If a person dies intestate, their estate is divided up under the rules of intestacy and a same sex partner has no legal claim. A LGBT patient wishing to leave their possessions to their partner must make their wishes clear in a will or have a Civil Partnership.

Living wills

A Living Will, or Advance Directive, is a set of advance instructions from a person of sound mind about their future medical care e.g. refusal or acceptance of treatments. This is not legally binding in the UK but most doctors will respect the wishes written in a living will. Unless a living will has been made, the family of origin can make decisions about medical intervention regardless of how long an LGBT couple have been together. In a Living Will the patient can specify a named person who they want to make decisions on their behalf should the need arise. This is another important means by which the role of the patient's partner/significant other can be validated.

Power of attorney

An LGBT patient can designate a partner or friend to act on their behalf if they become mentally incapable. Otherwise, this right passes directly to the legal next of kin.

Civil partnership

Under the Civil Partnership Act 2004, same sex couples can have the same legal rights as married couples.

Staff issues—sexual orientation in the team

How we feel about ourselves as sexual beings and how we function as a team in this area has a direct impact on the care we give patients and those close to them. Issues for hospice staff working with LGBT clients may include unresolved feelings in ourselves about sex and sexual preference or embarrassment over irrational responses. No one approaches this issue neutrally, everyone will bring their own experiences, feelings, views, and biases; when we are aware of our own feelings we are better able to attune to our patients' feelings.

Resources

- Terrence Higgins Trust: www.tht.org.uk. The UK's leading sexual health charity.
- London Friend: www.londonfriend.org.uk. Supports LGBT people across London and UK-wide via its two helplines: General LGBT helpline, 020 7837 3337; LGBT bereavement helpline, 020 7403 5969.
- Gendered Intelligence: www.genderedintelligence.co.uk. A UK-wide service for, and promoting the rights of, trans people.

References

Amnesty International. (2010). Jamaica: Submission to the UN Universal Periodic Review: Ninth session of the UPR Working Group of the Human Rights Council. New York: Amnesty International.

Bradford, J. and Ryan, C. (1988). *The National Lesbian Health Care Survey: Final Report.* Washington, DC: National Lesbian and Gay Health Foundation.

Bradford, J., Ryan, C., and Rothblum, E. D. (1994). National Lesbian Health Care Survey: Implications for mental health care. *Journal of Consulting and Clinical Psychology*, **62**: 228–42.

Colburn, K. and Malena, D. (1988). Bereavement issues for survivors of persons with AIDS: Coping with society's pressures. *Hospice Care*, 9/10.

Dean, L., Meyer I. H., Robinson, K., Sell, R. L., Sember, R., Silenzio, V. M. B., et al. (2000). Lesbian, gay, bisexual and transgender health. *Journal of the Gay and Lesbian Medical Association*, **4**(3): 102–51.

Department of Health. (1998). *The Health of the Nation: A Policy Assessed.* London: The Stationary Office.

Department of Health. (1999). *Saving Lives: Our Healthier Nation White Paper and Reducing Health Inequalities: An Action Report.* London: Department of Health.

Department of Health. (2004). *NICE Guidelines, 'Improving Supportive and Palliative Care for Adults with Cancer'.* London: The Stationery Office.

Doka, K. (ed.) (1989). *Disenfranchised Grief: Recognising Hidden Sorrow.* Massachusetts: Lexington Books.

Field, D., Hockey, J., and Small, N. (eds) (1997). *Death, Gender and Ethnicity.* London: Routledge.

Fisher, A., Vohr, F., and Wacker, M. (1996). Role of in-hospital palliative care service. *XI International Conference on AIDS*, Geneva, May.

Fitzpatrick, R., Dawson, J., Boulton, M., McLean, J., Hart, G., and Brookes, M. (1994). Perceptions of general practice among homosexual men. *British Journal of General Practice*, **44**: 80–2.

Flowers, P. and Buston, K. (2001). 'I was terrified of being different': Exploring gay men's accounts of growing-up in a heterosexist society. *Journal of Adolescence*, **24**: 51–65.

Harrison, N. (2000). Gay affirmative therapy: A critical analysis of the literature. *British Journal of Guidance and Counselling*, **28**(1): 37–53.

Kellerhouse, B. (1996). Voices from the front: The consequences of AIDS-related loss on six HIV negative gay men living in New York city. *XI International Conference on AIDS*, Geneva, May.

King, M. and McKeown, E. (2003). *Mental Health and Social Wellbeing of Gay Men, Lesbians and Bisexuals in England and Wales.* London: Mind.

King, M. and Nazareth, I. (2006). The health of people classified as lesbian, gay and bisexual attending family practitioners in London: A controlled study. *BMC Public Health*, **6**: 127.

King, M., McKeown, E., Warner, J., Ramsay, A., Johnson, K., Cort, C., et al. (2003). Mental health and quality of life of gay men and lesbians in England and Wales. *British Journal of psychiatry*, **183**: 552–8.

Oliviere, D., Hargreaves, R., and Monroe, B. (1998). *Good Practices in Palliative Care: A Psychosocial Perspective.* Aldershot, UK: Ashgate.

Plummer, K. (ed.) (1992). *Modern Homosexualities.* London: Routledge.

Savin-Williams, R. C. and Cohen, K. M. (eds) (1996). *The Lives of Lesbians, Gays, and Bisexuals: Children to Adults.* Fort Worth, TX: Harcourt Brace.

Sherr, L., Campbell, N., Crosier, A., and Meldrum, J. (1996). Suicide and AIDS: A report of the European Initiative. *XI International Conference on AIDS*, Geneva, May.

Sherr, L. (ed.) (1995). *Grief and AIDS* Chichester. London: John Wiley & Sons.

Weeks, J. (1995). *Invented Moralities: Sexual Values in an Age of Uncertainty.* Cambridge: Polity Press.

Chapter 21

Palliative care for prisoners

Mary Turner and Sheila Payne

Case examples

Paul

Paul (not his real name) was 39 when he was given a prison sentence in early 2009. Three months later he began coughing blood and was subsequently diagnosed with lung cancer. He received two courses of chemotherapy, after which he spent time recovering in the in-patient unit at Prison A, but was keen to return to the supportive community of his cellmates and staff at Prison B. Despite treatment, the tumour quickly doubled in size; Paul subsequently had palliative radiotherapy, but his prognosis was poor.

Paul discussed his preferred place of care with prison health care staff and his solicitor. He did not want to return to Prison A, but was not going to be able to stay at Prison B to die because it had no in-patient beds. He very much wanted to die at home, but his application for compassionate release was turned down, and refused again at appeal.

George

George (not his real name) was reaching the end of a long sentence when he was diagnosed in April 2008 with lung cancer. He was referred to the local hospice and attended day care, first as a prisoner and then following his release.

After George's release from prison, there was close collaboration between hospice day care staff, social services and George's probation officer, in the complex process of finding him somewhere suitable to live, acquiring furniture and making financial arrangements. Despite looking forward to independence, after the initial excitement of release he found it hard to live in the community. He was deteriorating physically, and felt isolated because he had no friends or family and his mobility was restricted. Hospice day care staff reported that he wished he had never been released but had instead stayed in prison to die.

Introduction

What is it like to die in prison, and how should dying prisoners be cared for? The two real life case examples presented above illustrate some of the complexities inherent in providing palliative care for prisoners; they also raise fundamental questions about how dying prisoners should be cared for in our society. In this chapter we will suggest that the prison population as a whole has to contend with multiple and severe disadvantages in terms of health, education, ageing, ethnicity, and disability compared with the rest of the population, and we will argue that consequently the needs of dying prisoners (and their families) for supportive and palliative care can be far greater than for other patients.

The prison population

Around 10 million people across the world are currently in prison, and there are huge variations in prison population rates between different countries (Walmsley, 2009). The United States has the highest rate in the world with 756 prisoners per 100,000 population, whilst India has one of the lowest rates with only 33 prisoners per 100,000 population. England and Wales has the highest rate in western Europe, with around 85,000 prisoners (153 per 100,000 population). Most prisoners are held as pre-trial detainees (remand prisoners) or as sentenced prisoners, while a minority are held for other reasons, for example in immigration removal centres.

Deaths in custody are relatively rare; in England and Wales in the year 2009–10 a total of 193 deaths in custody were reported, of which 116 (60%) were from natural causes (Prison and Probation Ombudsman, 2010). However, it is predicted that the prison population will continue to grow over the next few years (Ministry of Justice, 2009), with a probable corresponding rise in the number of anticipated deaths in prison. The need for good palliative care for prisoners is therefore likely to increase in the coming years.

The purpose of prison

It is important to consider the role of prison in any given society, because the purpose and philosophy behind different judicial systems may have a significant impact on the way dying prisoners are perceived and treated. Justice systems vary considerably across the world; some countries have extremely punitive systems whilst others adopt a more liberal stance. In some countries greater emphasis is placed on punishment (especially, it could be argued, those countries that employ the death penalty as the ultimate sanction). Indeed, the element of punishment is present in any system, even if only at the level of depriving people of their liberty. In some countries however, such as Australia, the focus is on the rehabilitation of offenders:

> A basic question needs answering—what is the use of a prison system which returns an offender to the community the same if not worse than when he or she entered prison? The philosophy in most modern prisons systems is to try and change the behaviour of offenders by developing in them skills which see all people live in the community without resorting to crime. (Government of South Australia, 2010)

Prisons also exist to protect the public. Her Majesty's Prison Service for England and Wales states on its website that it protects the public by holding prisoners securely and reducing the risk of re-offending; it also provides 'safe and well-ordered establishments in which we treat prisoners humanely, decently and lawfully' (HMPS, 2010).

A closer look at prisoners

So far we have presented some facts and figures to provide an overview of the prison population. But who are the people confined in our prisons? To begin with, the vast majority are male; in England and Wales, men constitute 95% of the prison population, and women only 5% (Ministry of Justice, 2010). In addition, a disproportionate number of prisoners are from minority ethnic groups. Around 10% of the UK population is from minority ethnic backgrounds, yet a report by Nacro (the crime reduction charity in England and Wales) states that prisoners from minority ethnic groups account for 21% of the male prison population and 26% of the female prison population (Nacro, 2003); this pattern is repeated in other countries, including the US.

The Prison Reform Trust (2010) estimates that up to 30% of prisoners have learning disabilities or difficulties that interfere with their ability to cope with the criminal justice system; prisoners with learning disabilities have been shown to be the least likely to know when their parole or release date was, to ask if they did not understand something, or to know what to do if they felt unwell. A disproportionate number of prisoners are also at a disadvantage because of poor educational attainment; 48% of prisoners are at or below the level expected of an 11-year-old in reading, and 82% in writing.

In addition, it is estimated that 70% of the prison population have two or more diagnosed mental illnesses (the most common of which is depression). Many prisoners have to contend with multiple health and social problems; for example, a high proportion of prisoners from minority ethnic groups also have mental health problems. A report by Nacro (2007) states that 'recent figures show that black communities are over 40% more likely than average to be referred to mental health services through the criminal justice system' (p. 1). It is therefore perhaps not surprising that one systematic review (Harris, Hek, et al., 2006) found that prisoners are more likely to have suffered some form of social exclusion compared with the rest of society.

Although the prison population is predominantly made up of younger people, the average age of prisoners is rising, and the number of older prisoners is increasing (Linder and Meyers, 2007). There are specific issues to be considered in relation to age and ageing in prisons. At the turn of the twenty-first century, the average age of death for the whole population in England and Wales was 73.2 years for men and 79.4 years for women. In stark contrast to these figures, the average age of male prisoners who died from natural causes between 2004 and 2010 was 56, whilst for females it was only 47 (Prison and Probation Ombudsman, 2010). The most common cause of these natural deaths was heart disease, followed by cancer. Even taking into account the relatively small numbers of individuals involved, and recognizing that only a small proportion of people in their seventies and eighties are in prison, these figures nevertheless indicate that prison has an adverse effect on health. It has also been suggested that prison causes premature ageing; some older prisoners are believed to have a physical health status of 10 years older than their contemporaries in the rest of society (Prison Reform Trust, 2008). Older prisoners also frequently have to deal with multiple health problems; one study found that 85% of older prisoners (over 60 years of age) had one or more major illnesses, the most common of which were psychiatric, cardiovascular, musculoskeletal, and respiratory (Fazel, Hope, et al., 2001).

It has been argued that life expectancy is shorter amongst prisoners because they take less exercise, smoke more and have a poorer diet than most of the population.

Frances Crook, Director of the Howard League for Penal Reform, contends that prison is used as a 'dumping ground' for the mentally ill, poor and dispossessed, stating that:

> People arrive in prison having a history of poor mental and physical health. Rather than treating their problems sensibly, we are using prison to sweep them away from public view, thus shortening their already troubled lives. Prison is an expensive way of hastening the death of poor people. (Crook, 2010)

Organization of health services in prisons

In 2004 prison health care in England and Wales was transferred from prison control to the National Health Service, and services and staff are now provided in each prison and managed by local Primary Care Trusts. This has had the benefit of streamlining services and promoting the development of good working relationships between staff inside and outside of the prisons.

In 2008, a strategy for end of life care in England and Wales was published by the Department of Health, which contains a clear recommendation that end of life care should be available to all who need it, regardless of diagnosis, social factors, or care settings. The strategy explicitly identifies prisons as one area where attention needs to be paid to the provision of end of life care (Department of Health, 2008). A study undertaken in 2009 to evaluate the provision of end of life care services in prisons in the north-west of England found some evidence that geographical factors may influence the provision of palliative care for prisoners; prisons geographically close to hospices or other palliative care services appeared to have made more progress in this area that those further afield (Turner, Payne, et al., 2010). As part of the same study, prison health care staff were asked to identify barriers to delivering good end of life care. The most frequently cited barriers were the environment, resources and equipment. Even resources such as continence materials, which are commonly available to other dying patients in the community, are often difficult to obtain in prisons. The physical environment in some prisons can also present specific challenges; even if equipment such as hospital beds are available, some older prison buildings are not suitable for their use because the cells are too small or because numerous steps make access impossible. One prison in the north-west of England, for example, is housed in a castle that dates back to the twelfth century; this is a listed building owned by English Heritage, so alterations, such as creating disabled access, are simply not possible.

Compassionate release

The case example of Paul highlights the issue of place of care at the end of life, and raises questions about whether or not prisoners should be released early on compassionate grounds. The issue of compassionate release is controversial, particularly in the aftermath of the high-profile releases in 2009 of Abdelbaset Ali al-Megrahi (the 'Lockerbie Bomber') and Ronnie Biggs (the 'Great Train Robber'), both of whom went on to live long after the predicted three months that allowed them to fulfil the criteria for compassionate release (Turner, Barbarachild, et al., 2009). Many people, including relatives of people who died at Lockerbie, believe that criminals do not deserve compassion, even at the end of life. The Prison and Probation Ombudsman

(2010), however, recommends that 'releasing terminally ill prisoners on compassionate grounds should be the norm unless security factors militate against it' (p. 14). In the case of Paul, although he was refused compassionate release, the Governor at his prison allowed him home on compassionate leave, where he died with his family around him.

Impact on prisoners' families

The amount of compassion and support shown to dying prisoners and their families is likely to have an effect on families that may last for many years into their bereavement. Even in cases where compassionate release is not possible, there are many ways in which compassion can be shown. For example, allowing prison officers not to wear uniform when escorting dying prisoners to hospital or hospice appointments affords the prisoner a degree of dignity which may be particularly valued by family members. Family members may also need the support of their relative who is in prison when they themselves are ill and dying. However, in England and Wales, in order to be allowed to visit dying family members, prisoners have to undergo rigorous assessment before approval for release on temporary licence can be granted by the Governor or another authorized senior manager, and not all prisoners are eligible for temporary release.

It is also important that families are supported following the death of a prisoner, as all deaths in custody in the UK are subject to both Coroner's Inquest and independent investigation by the Prisons and Probation Ombudsman. A survey of bereaved families conducted by the Prisons and Probation Ombudsman (Gauge, 2010) showed that most families appreciated the support provided by the Family Liaison Officers in the Ombudsman's office, but there were concerns about the time taken to complete the investigations. Prisoners' families and friends are likely to have specific needs in relation to their bereavement and may experience complex grieving processes. The stigma attached to being in prison may make it difficult for bereaved families to feel they can access local or national bereavement support services, and indeed services that are accustomed to supporting those whose relatives died at home or in a hospice might struggle to meet the specific needs of prisoners' families.

It is also worth remembering that when death occurs in prison, particularly when the individual has served a long sentence, other prisoners may feel the loss keenly and need support to cope with their bereavement. The case example of George highlights the importance of friendships between prisoners; when George was released, he could no longer access the social support that had been available to him in prison.

Staff

To date very little research has been undertaken in the field of palliative care for prisoners. However, in a useful paper, Crawley (2005) identifies the concept of 'institutional thoughtlessness', which refers to the idea that all prisoners should be treated the same, and nobody deserves any special treatment regardless of whether they are old, disabled, or dying. Where the prevailing culture in prison is that the prisoners are there to be punished, it is easy to see how institutional thoughtlessness can become the norm for staff. It is also important to consider the experiences of prison officers in relation to death; a significant proportion of deaths in prison are the result of suicide or other violent acts, and prison officers are first on the scene in these extremely harrowing situations. It is hardly surprising therefore if prison officers perceive death in prison as something to be avoided rather than planned for. There is a clear need for adequate staff support, as well as education and training around end of life care, if dying prisoners are to receive high quality palliative care.

Conclusion

There is mounting evidence that end of life care for prisoners is beginning to improve both in the UK and elsewhere. In 2007, Europe's first 'pensioners only prison' opened in Singen in Germany, with purpose-built cells designed to accommodate older prisoners with walking frames and wheelchairs. In the UK, examples of good practice are being identified and shared, and staff from both inside and outside prisons are working together to promote mutual learning and ultimately improve care. For example, in one area in north-west England, palliative care staff from one hospice have established regular meetings with health care staff from three local prisons to discuss and plan the care of dying prisoners (Turner, Payne, et al., 2010). A key element of good practice is flexibility and responsiveness; this is exemplified in the case of Paul. The first time Paul was transferred to the in-patient unit in Prison A, following a day of chemotherapy treatment, it took several hours for him to get into a bed because he had to go through Prison A's security and reception procedures; his property did not arrive from the hospital until three days later when he was packing up to go back to Prison B, so whilst he was in Prison A he did not even have the book he had been reading. However, these problems were recognized and acknowledged by the Governors of both prisons, prison health care staff, and hospital staff, who all worked hard to ensure that the second time he had treatment and was transferred to Prison A the whole process was managed much more smoothly.

The Prisons and Probation Ombudsman (2010) believes that the quality of palliative care services in prisons has improved significantly since 2004, and he regards this as a 'substantial achievement'. However, there is more work to be done. We have shown that dying prisoners and their families face multiple challenges and are often disadvantaged in myriad ways. Given the increasing and ageing prison population, it is clear that initiatives to improve palliative care for dying prisoners will need to continue to develop over the coming years.

> How we care for the dying is an indicator of how we care for all sick and vulnerable people. It is a measure of society as a whole . . . (Department of Health, 2008: 10)

Resources

- Prisons and Probation Ombudsman (independent ombudsman who investigates the complaints of prisoners and probationers): www.ppo.gov.uk.
- Nacro (the crime reduction charity in England and Wales): www.nacro.org.uk.

◆ Prison Reform Trust (works to ensure prisons are just, humane and effective): www.prisonreformtrust.org.uk.

References

Crawley, E. (2005). Surviving the prison experience? Imprisonment and elderly men. *Prison Service Journal*, **160**: 9–10.

Crook, F. (2010). Prison hastens death for poor (letter to the editor). *Observer*, Sunday 15 August.

Department of Health. (2008). *End of Life Care Strategy—Promoting High Quality Care for all Adults at the End of Life*. London: Department of Health.

Fazel, S., Hope, T., O'Donnell, I., Piper, M., and Jacoby, R. (2001). Health of elderly male prisoners: Worse than the general population, worse than younger prisoners. *Age and Ageing*, **30**: 403–7.

Gauge, S. (2010). *Prisons and Probation Ombudsman Bereaved Families' Feedback Survey 2009*. Available from www.ppo.gov.uk/docs/PPO_Bereaved_families_report_2009.pdf.

Government of South Australia. (2010). Prison and Prisoner Management website. Available at: www.corrections.sa.gov.au/prisons. Accessed 11 May 2010.

Harris, F., Hek, G., and Condon, L. (2006). Health needs of prisoners in England and Wales: The implications for prison healthcare of gender, age and ethnicity. *Health and Social Care in the Community*, **15**(1): 56–66.

Her Majesty's Prison Service. (2010). Available from: www.hmprisonservice.gov.uk/abouttheservice/statementofpurpose/. Accessed 22 Sept. 2010.

Linder, J. F. and Meyers, F. J. (2007). Palliative care for prison inmates: 'Don't let me die in prison'. *Journal of the American Medical Association*, **298**(8): 894–901.

Ministry of Justice. (2009). *Prison Population Projections 2009–2015: England and Wales*. London: Ministry of Justice.

Ministry of Justice. (2010). *Prison Population and Accommodation Briefing for 17th September 2010*. Available from: www.hmprisonservice.gov.uk/resourcecentre/publicationsdocuments/index.asp?cat=85. Accessed 22 September 2010.

Nacro. (2003). *Race and Prisons: Where Are We Now?* London: Nacro. Available from: www.nacro.org.uk/data/files/nacro-2008122309-299.pdf. Accessed 21 Sept. 2010.

Nacro. (2007). *Policy Briefing: Black Communities, Mental Health and the Criminal Justice System*. Available from: www.nacro.org.uk/data/files/nacro-2007052400-271.pdf. Accessed 21 Sept. 2010.

Prison and Probation Ombudsman. (2010). *Annual Report 2009–2010*. London: Prison and Probation Ombudsman for England and Wales.

Prison Reform Trust. (2008). *Doing Time: The Experiences and Needs of Older People in Prison*. London: Prison Reform Trust.

Prison Reform Trust. (2010). Available at: www.prisonreformtrust.org.uk/. Accessed 22 Sept. 2010.

Turner, M., Barbarachild, Z., Kidd, H., and Payne, S. (2009). How notorious do dying prisoners need to be to receive high quality end-of-life care? *International Journal of Palliative Nursing*, **15**(10): 472–3.

Turner, M., Payne, S., and Barbarachild, Z. (2010). Care or custody? An evaluation of palliative care in prisons in North West England. *Palliative Medicine* **25**(4): 370–7.

Walmsley, R. (2009). *World Prison Population List (Eighth Edition)*. International Centre for Prison Studies, King's College London. Available from: www.kcl.ac.uk/depsta/law/research/icps/downloads/wppl-8th_41.pdf. Accessed 21 Sept. 2010.

Chapter 22

Bereavement—a world of difference

Orla Keegan

This chapter will set out current thinking on bereavement, grief, and loss, identifying the different influences on their construction. It will then go on to review how points in the life cycle, aspects of life circumstances and of death circumstances contribute to different experiences of grief, and ultimately bereavement supports.

Different perspectives on bereavement

Current thinking about bereavement is characterized by sensitivity to individual difference and variety in ways of grieving. The previously dominant views are giving way to newer perspectives which seek to accommodate a variety of bereavement experiences (Genevro, Marshall, et al. 2004; Stroebe, Hannson, et al., 2008). Specifically, there has been a move away from prescriptive, staged frameworks (Kubler-Ross, 1970) to models which are more fluid, coping-oriented, and comprehensive (Stroebe and Schut, 1999) and to those which see a role for others in supporting sense-making or meaning-making processes (Neimeyer, 2000). These social reconstruction models hold that grief is what we make it, a new chapter but part of our ongoing story, a different life.

A move from solely 'pathology' focused bereavement models is evident, towards those identifying resilience, growth and strength coming out of the pain associated with loss (Bonnanno, 2009; Machin, 2007). The accumulation of scientific work allows us to trace the real and differential health outcomes associated with (if not caused by) bereavement—the early mortality risk factors for widowed men for example, and a range of negative physical and mental health issues for men and women (Stroebe et al., 2007) as well as criteria for diagnosing the smaller proportions of people who develop more serious complications or 'prolonged grief' (Prigerson et al., 2009).

Discipline-specific inquiry, including medical, social and psychological lenses underpin different descriptions of and explanations for the grief experience. Each approach takes a different relative emphasis to the ultimate nature of grief, its measurement, and potential treatment. Social and psychological models dominate the literature with the physiological and cultural determinants requiring more attention (Stroebe et al., 2008) and sociological models for grief's regulation beyond the initial death and funeral disappointingly lacking (Ribbens-McCarthy, 2006).

Different viewpoints have real implications. Silverman (2000a) uncovers the different perspectives taken by researchers and clinicians in the area of bereavement, concluding that the two sectors rarely meet and there may be much to be gained by actively promoting these discussions. She describes individually-focused clinicians, working with clients' problems to deadlines with quick turnarounds, removed and separate from researchers focusing on group trends, with long-term goals and often uninvolved in the application of their findings. The agendas are illustrated as set separately, there is some overlap at data collection phases, and little conversing after that, including in the interpretation of research findings. Bridging these different worlds may help to address the lag in the dissemination and adoption of newer grief models and interventions and promote relevant investigation (Sandler et al., 2005).

Different grief experiences

Grief is not a single phenomenon and there are several major dimensions which lend viewpoints for understanding variety in grief experiences—these include different lifecycle stages, different modes of death, and different social contexts.

Grief through the lifecycle

In a very rudimentary way grief will be experienced through the developmental status of the griever, for example, a child's experience of grief and his/her mourning is limited and constrained by cognitive development and the degree to which the permanence of separation is understood. The infant or toddler's experience of grief can be an almost physical yearning, qualitatively different to the younger child's ability to understand 'gone', and the physical qualities of death as a state, but not the time dimension and irreversibility of death (Silverman, 2000b).

During adolescence the competing drives for independence and security can make for a difficult loss experience. A death can set the adolescent further apart from peers and from other family members and making sense of a shattering change in family structure through loss of a parent or loss of a sibling coinciding with the adolescent's attempts to develop their own sense of identity (Balk and Corr, 2009).

It could be argued that the middle adult years are the neglected years when it comes to what is known about grief, despite the fact that most adults become orphaned at this point. The bereavement literature yields a preponderance of research on the state of widowhood, on older age and on children's grief but relatively little on bereavement experienced in middle age (Walter and McCoyd, 2009).

Loss in older age is often considered an inevitability; however there are two potential interpretations of the experience of loss in older age, on what may make it different. One is that cumulative loss and the natural order inoculates the griever, the opposing view is that loss of long standing, important and supportive relationships takes a greater toll. The important prospective, longitudinal study of older couples conducted by Bonanno and his colleagues (2002) makes a point which at first appears deceptively simple—that older people are not a homogenous group. 'Older people' are defined by difference, they meet loss and bereavement from different starting points and they cope in different ways. The study identifies an expected (but small) cohort of older people whose mental health deteriorates following spousal bereavement and gradually restores. However, a substantially larger proportion are identified whose main characteristic is resilience, their mental health status barely impacted by 6 months and returning to normal relatively quickly following the loss. Two other trends were discerned,—those whose depression lifted following a death, and those (a small proportion) who, depressed before the death, remained so.

Different lives: different losses

Doka (2002) has done the world of grief work an important service by defining the term 'disenfranchised grief'. It is a concept predicated on difference, and on questioning the assumptions around capacity and rights to grieve. In the past here have been dominant and often harsh societal assumptions which had impacts on certain sectors of society. Amongst these assumptions were that some groups do not experience grief (e.g. young children, intellectually disabled people) or that some losses simply do not hurt (e.g. death of an estranged spouse). Finally, the dominance of a majority view meant that the different experiences of some groups were simply hidden and some losses were invisible where relationships were not known about or experiences were not shared, e.g. gay and lesbian relationships (Glackin and Higgins, 2008), relinquishing/natural mothers in adoption. Green and Grant (2008) highlight the moral dimension of judgement which can underpin disenfranchised grief.

The fundamentally different way of being in the world that is 'gender' is another important difference in thinking about grief. Gender is a construct that is played out in the world, subtle and not so subtle pressure comes to bear on men and women that suggests the most appropriate ways of experiencing, and of displaying grief. Walter (1999) was amongst the first to identify the 'feminization' of grief support arguing that the counselling, emotion-focused model of bereavement dominates to the exclusion of other experiences and support structures. Martin and Doka (2000) identifying 'styles' of grief, describe a range of memorializing, task centred and problem solving activities such as fundraising, lobbying, working and 'getting on', which they term 'instrumental' and valid means of grieving. Whether grief is experienced differently by men and women is debatable, what is a feature of the difference is the dominance of display rules and expectations that people use, for themselves, and for each other. The work of Bennett (2007) demonstrates the masculine pressures to be strong, independent and a provider including in bereavement—the masculine hegemony which mitigates against emotional responses, particularly in public. Where gender dynamics and different experiences and/or styles of grieving become particularly important is when couples are bereaved through the death of a child (Riches and Dawson, 2000).

Finally, some contexts allow us to make grief invisible, to limit its reach. The world of work for example is where the majority of the population spend the majority of their lives. However, the objective design of the commercial contract implies that people divide their emotional time just as they divide their work/non-work hours. A number of recent initiatives have contested this seeking to reorient the workplace culture and maximizing the value placed on employees. Charles-Edwards' (2000) emotionally intelligent book on this topic begins with deconstructing the 'least said soonest mended' adage. He places care within the responsibilities of organizations and the people within them by identifying comfort with talking about death and bereavement as the first step. In Ireland a Grief and Work Policy was launched giving guidance on some of the practical and training initiatives workplaces can engage in to promote flexibility and understanding (McGuinness, 2007).

Different deaths: different losses

The wider healthcare and sociological literature increasingly considers the 'good death', as an aspiration for the Western population—the best way to die is at home, surrounded by those you love and free from pain. This death, it is concluded, will serve the dying and the bereaved and much of the policy set out in the UK and elsewhere seeks to maximize choice and the comfortable death (e.g. Department of Health, 2009).

The reality of death and dying is very different in 2011. Much of the world lives and dies in poverty, with life expectancy starkly contrasting across the regions of the world, favouring resource rich over resource poor countries (World Health Organization, 2008). Chronic health issues and institutional death in old age characterizes the majority death in western Europe (Davies and Higginson, 2004). Sudden, accidental and suicide deaths continue to make up an increasing proportion of death statistics. Some of these due to their suddenness/unexpectedness, combined with a potential for trauma, may influence the shape of grief (Currier, Holland, et al., 2006).

However the cause and nature of a death is only one factor. While some have demonstrated that those deaths with a trauma potential (e.g. suicide and homicide) are most intense and may lead to difficulties in adjusting (Hogan et al., 2001; Gamino et al., 2009), others stress the importance of looking at the full complexity of personal, relationship and other issues (Stroebe, Folkman, et al., 2006).

Deaths in the military

Many of the dimensions of difference considered earlier in this chapter are relevant to deaths in the armed forces. Bereavement in the military context takes on a different shape for a number of reasons, most of them associated with the 'cultural script' of army life and the foregrounding of the possibility of dying. Ben-Ari (2005) describes this script as involving 'death in combat-related activities within publicly accepted conflicts of young, unattached men and (rarely) women; retrieval of the whole body or all of its parts; the conduct of a full military funeral and official commemorations accompanied by informal rites of remembering (within the soldiers' unit); and some kind of psychological resolution for kith and kin'.

Echoes of such a script are evident where Cawkhill (2009) describes the degree of formal grief and bereavement support through the armed forces in the UK, that formalization being apparent in the naming of relevant roles who interact with family— the 'Casualty Notifying' officer, the 'Visiting Officer' for up to a year after a death.

Death in the army is both expected, in that the general possibility of dying is planned for, and unexpected in the actual events preceding and causing death. Violence and trauma are features of death in combat, as is the loss of young soldiers. These young deaths however, are connected to a meaning unit of 'noble cause' and 'sacrifice' and these are assumed in some way to support the bereaved families and to provide comfort (Ben-Ari, 2005). The extent to which those meaning frameworks actually ameliorate the loss is not established however. In addition, given the political and domestic public opposition to certain wars and involvement in armed conflict, there is no certainty that the full backing of a society is behind the cause, and ultimately the sacrifice of these soldiers. Consequently the wider help and support available to army families is unconsidered and unexplored in recent literature.

Outside of combat-related mortality large proportions of service men (and fewer women) die through accident, illness and injury at home and on service. Stigma and disenfranchisement may be an experience for families in some circumstances, such as suicide. Armed forces internationally are coming to terms with their responsibilities to staff and the additional suicide risk factors in military life including military deployment as a stressful life event, traumatic brain injury, and post-traumatic stress disorder (Martin et al., 2009). Recognizing some challenges, the Mental Health America Foundation sponsors a programme to overcome stigma around suicide in the armed forces. Amongst its campaigns is a petition to seek equal honours (e.g. a condolence letter from the president) to be sent to army families bereaved through the suicide of their soldier relative. In the United Kingdom new developments have seen Ministry of Defence systems link to community and voluntary organizations such as Cruse Bereavement Care to provide support and training (Cawkhill, 2009).

Grief support systems—appropriate support meeting different needs

Outlined above are some of the wide range of variables that may impact on grief and bereavement, on how individuals experience it, how societies interpret and regulate it, and on how helping structures are organized. Underpinning the discussion is the assumption that *understanding grief* helps to support it.

In order to accommodate difference, supports need to be flexible, accessible and appropriate—and not always organized. Formal and organized bereavement supports in voluntary, community, and health settings have grown in responsive and useful ways. However, it could be argued that at the same time spontaneous support systems of neighbourhood, parish, and family have declined and fragmented, eroding the natural base for grief support. Kellehear's (2005) 'compassionate cities' framework describes a system wide approach to care at the end of life, including bereavement care. It proposes a change of attitude beginning with awareness-raising and the re-adjustment of systems—for example, of work structures, to accommodate caring responsibilities of employees, of environments such as gardens and public spaces for bereaved people in an accepted and normalized way. The health-promoting approach he outlines does more than accommodate difference; it expects it and responds to it through natural, human care.

The evidence based models for levels of bereavement service in cancer and palliative care (NICE, 2004) outline a similar approach by identifying ascending components to bereavement care where component one acknowledges the role of natural support networks, of available, up-to-date and accurate information on bereavement. This work is further developed in work commissioned by the National Office for Suicide Prevention in Ireland where an underpinning capacity-development foundation of education and awareness-raising is proposed for comprehensive bereavement care (Petrus Consulting et al., 2008).

When it comes to accessing more formal volunteer or health-related services, differences in literacy, mobility, and existing social support all have implications for how a person might investigate and find out about such supports, and how they might actually access them. In addition there is arguably further inequity in access to bereavement care—few supports are domiciliary, there is little variety in models (with the individual counselling model remaining dominant) and routes ranging from self-referral to professional referral are ad hoc.

Formal bereavement support (including volunteer-based befriending, listening, and counselling services; professional counselling services and psychological and therapeutic supports) has increasingly been criticized for lacking a sound evidence base. The mechanisms by which services are accessed and referred to are also coming under scrutiny—there is little to suggest that primary/universal services offered to *all* bereaved make a difference to the intensity, duration, or quality of grief experience. Services offered more selectively (secondary supports) to those deemed 'at risk' have shown modest, if not sustained, benefits; most evidence points to an impact for the formal therapeutic bereavement interventions (tertiary or indicated services) which are made available to those who are symptomatic or experiencing real complications through grief (Schut and Stroebe, 2005; Currier, Neimeyer, et al., 2008).

Some of the difficulties in establishing the effectiveness of bereavement support reflect the very variety and difference in bereavement experience outlined in this chapter. At the same time services are often bound together by single themes—the nature of the relationship, e.g. parents' support, the type of death, e.g. suicide, or accessed through single routes, e.g. hospice bereavement supports for hospice deaths, hospital services for hospital deaths. The extent to which these supports link to each other is often limited (Field, Payne, et al., 2007). Cawkhill's description of the Bereavement Care Pathways project linking NHS, community and military amongst others is an ambitious exception (Cawkhill, 2009).

An argument remains as to how best to provide bereavement care as an integrated activity, part of normal caring networks, ascending to higher levels of support when needed. While the problem associated with focusing on difference may lead to a fragmented service landscape, lifecycle, and community development models hold some integrating promise as we move into the future.

Resources

- General public information about bereavement
  www.bbc.co.uk/health/emotional_health/bereavement/
- Example of Bereavement Services for military families (England)
  www.crusebereavementcare.org.uk/Military.html
- Academic collection of chapters outlining current understanding of grief, influences on bereavement, and a range of interventions.
- Stroebe, M. S., Hansson, R. O., Schut, H., and Stroebe, W. (2008). *Handbook of Bereavement Research and Practice: Advances in theory and intervention.* Washington, DC: APA.

References

Balk, D. and Corr, C. (2009). *Adolescent Encounters with Death, Bereavement, and Coping.* New York: Springer Publishing.

Ben-Ari, E. (2005). Epilogue: A good military death. *Armed Forces and Society*, **31**(4): 651–64.

Bennett, K. (2007). 'No sissy stuff': Towards a theory of masculinity and emotional expression in older widowed men. *Journal of Aging Studies*, **21**: 347–56.

Bonanno, G. A., Wortman, C. B., Lehman, D. R., Tweed, R. G., Haring, M., Sonnega, J., et al. (2002). Resilience to loss and chronic grief: A prospective study from preloss to 18-months postloss. *Journal of Personal and Social Psychology*, **83**(5): 1150–64.

Bonanno, G. (2009). *The Other Side of Sadness: What the New Science of Bereavement Tells Us about Life After Loss.* New York: Basic Books.

Cawkill, P. (2009). Death in the armed forces: Casualty notification and bereavement support in the UK military. *Bereavement Care*, **28**(2): 25–30.

Charles-Edwards, D. (2000). *Bereavement at Work: A Practical Guide.* London: Duckworth.

Currier, J. M., Neimeyer, R. A., and Berman, J. S. (2008). The effectiveness of psychotherapeutic interventions for bereaved persons: A comprehensive quantitative review. *Psychological Bulletin*, **134**(5): 648–61.

Currier, J., Holland, J., and Neimeyer, R. (2006). Sense-making, grief, and the experience of violent loss: Toward a mediational model. *Death Studies*, **30**(5): 403–28.

Davies, E. and Higginson, I. (eds) (2004). *Palliative Care: The Solid Facts.* Denmark: World Health Organization.

Department of Health. (2009). *End of Life Care Strategy: First Annual Report.* London: Department of Health.

Doka, K. (ed.) (2002). *Disenfranchised Grief: New Directions, Challenges and Strategies for Practice.* Champaign, IL: Research Press.

Field, D. Payne, S., Relf, M., and Reid, D. (2007). Some issues in the provision of adult bereavement support by UK hospices. *Social Science & Medicine*, **64**(2): 428–38.

Gamino, L. A., Sewell, K. W., Hogan, N. S., and Mason S. L. (2009). Who needs grief counselling? A report from the Scott & White Grief Study. *Omega*, **60**(3): 199–223.

Genevro, J. L., Marshall, T., and Miller, T. (2004). Report on bereavement and grief research. *Death Studies*, **28**(6): 491–575.

Glackin, M. and Higgins, A. (2008). The grief experience of same-sex couples within an Irish context: Tacit acknowledgement. *International Journal of Palliative Nursing*, **14**(6): 297–302.

Green, L. and Grant, V. (2008). Gagged grief and beleaguered bereavements? An analysis of multidisciplinary theory and research relating to same sex partnership bereavement. *Sexualities*, **11**(3): 275–300.

Hogan, N. S., Greenfield, D. B., and Schmidt, L. A. (2001). Development and validation of the Hogan Grief Reaction Checklist. *Death Studies*, **25**(1): 1–32.

Kellehear, A. (2005). *Compassionate Cities: Public Health and End of Life Care.* New York: Routledge.

Kubler-Ross, E. (1970). *On Death and Dying.* London: Tavistock.

Machin, L. (2007). Resilience and bereavement: Part 1, In B. Monroe and D. Oliviere(eds), *Resilience in Palliative Care: Achievement in Adversity.* Oxford: Oxford University Press.

Martin, T. L. and Doka, K. J. (2000). *Men Don't Cry . . . Women Do: Transcending Gender Stereotypes of Grief.* Philadelphia: Brunner-Mazel.

Martin, J., Ghahramanlou-Holloway, M., Lou, K., and Tucciarone, P. (2009). A comparative review of U.S. military and civilian suicide behaviour: Implications for OEF/OIF suicide prevention efforts. *Journal of Mental Health Counselling*, **31**(2): 101–18.

McGuinness, B. (2007). *Grief at Work: Developing a Policy on Bereavement in the Workplace.* Dublin: Irish Hospice Foundation.

Mental Health America. Operation Healthy Reunions. Available at www.nmha.org/reunions/resources.cfm. Accessed 24 Sept. 2010.

National Institute for Clinical Excellence. (2004). *Supportive and Palliative Care for Cancer with Adults* [ONLINE]. Available from: www.nice.org.uk/page.aspx?o=csgsp. Accessed Jan. 2010.

Neimeyer, R. (2000). *Meaning Reconstruction and the Experience of Loss.* Washington, DC: APA.

Petrus Consulting, Bates, U., Jordan, N., Malone, K., Monahan, E., O'Connor, S., and Tiernan, E. (2008). *Review of General Bereavement Support and Specific Services Available Following Suicide Review.* Dublin: National Office for Suicide Prevention.

Prigerson, H. G., Horowitz, M. J., Jacobs, S. C., Parkes, C. M., Aslan, M., Gooedkin, K., et al. (2009). Prolonged grief disorder: Psychometric validation of criteria proposed for DSM-V and ICD-11. *PLoS Med*, **6**(8): e1000121.

Ribbens-McCarthy, J. (2006). *Young People's Experiences of Loss and Bereavement: Towards an Inter-disciplinary Approach.* Buckingham, UK: Open University Press.

Riches, G. and Dawson, P. (2000). *An Intimate Loneliness: Supporting Bereaved Parents and Siblings.* Buckingham, UK: Open University Press.

Sandler, I., Balk, D., Jordan, J., Kennedy, C., Nadeau, J., and Shapiro, E. (2005). Bridging the gap between research and practice in bereavement: Report from the Center for the Advancement of Health. *Death Studies*, **29**(2): 93–122.

Schut, H. and Stroebe, M. S. (2005). Interventions to enhance adaptation to bereavement. *Journal of Palliative Medicine*, **8**(Suppl. 1): S140–7.

Silverman, P. R. (2000a). Research, clinical practice, and the human experience: Putting the pieces together. *Death Studies*, **24**(6): 469–78.

Silverman, P. R. (2000b). *Never Too Young to Know: Death in Children's Lives.* Oxford: Oxford University Press.

Stroebe, M. S. and Schut, H. (1999). The dual process model of coping with bereavement: Rationale and description. *Death Studies*, **23**: 197–224.

Stroebe, M. S., Folkman, S., Hansson, R., and Schut, H. (2006). The prediction of bereavement outcome: Development of an integrative risk factor framework. *Social Science & Medicine*, **63**(9): 2440–51.

Stroebe, M. S., Schut, H., and Stroebe, W. (2007). Health outcomes of bereavement. *The Lancet*, **370**(9603): 1960–73.

Stroebe, M. S., Hansson, R. O., Schut, H., and Stroebe, W. (2008). *Handbook of Bereavement Research and Practice: Advances in Theory and Intervention.* Washington, DC: APA.

Walter, C. A. and McCoyd, J. L. M. (2009). *Grief and Loss Across the Lifespan: A Biopsychosocial Perspective.* Danvers, MA: Springer Publishing.

Walter, T. (1999). *On Bereavement: The Culture of Grief.* Buckinghamshire, UK: Open University Press.

World Health Organization. (2008). *Life Tables for WHO Member States.* www.who.int/healthinfo/statistics/mortality_life_tables/en/.

Afterword

Mike Richards

National Clinical Director for Cancer and End of Life Care

One of the benefits of being invited to write an 'afterword' is that I have had the privilege of reading the preceding chapters prior to publication. I will start by congratulating the editors both on tackling such an important topic as death, dying, and social differences and on assembling such an excellent panel of experts to write individual chapters. I would also like to congratulate the chapter authors for the way in which they have combined knowledge and academic rigour with compassion for the groups of people they are writing about.

Some readers will have followed a logical order by starting at the beginning of this book and working forwards. They will already have come to their conclusions about the topics and chapters that gave them the greatest new insights. Other readers (and I am one) have a tendency to start by opening a book towards the end and then picking and choosing which chapters to read. These readers have a treat in store!

For me, a recurring highlight in reading the various contributions to this book has been the use of personal stories or case histories of people approaching the end of life to introduce key issues which are then discussed. These include Nicole, a 66-year-old with cerebral palsy who was desperately keen to stay at home (Chapter 8); Simon, an Australian teenager who decided to travel to England when he knew he had terminal cancer (Chapter 11); Pete Carpenter, with severe intellectual disabilities (Chapter 12); Deborah, a 42-year-old with long-standing paranoid schizophrenia (Chapter 13); JW, a 63-year-old Traveller (Chapter 16); several asylum seekers or refugees (Chapter 17); Jon, who was gay, Marie who was bisexual, and Fiona who was a lesbian (Chapter 20), and two prisoners, Paul and George (Chapter 21).

Each of these stories and the accompanying wealth of information will be of great interest to a wide range of professionals working the field of palliative or end of life care. I learned new information from almost every chapter. To give just two examples, although I was aware that death at home can be unacceptable to some travelling people, I was not aware that Roma believe that the lower half of the body is less pure than the upper half, which has implications for health care workers washing Roma patients. I was also unaware of the average age of people dying from natural causes in prisons (56 for men and 47 for women).

As might be expected I have also read the book from the perspective of a policy-maker committed to improving the quality of end of life care for everyone approaching the end of life and for reducing inequalities in access to high-quality care. Several of the contributors to this book have made reference to the End of Life Care Strategy (2008) and in particular to the statement 'How we care for the dying is an indicator of how we care for all sick and vulnerable people. It is a measure of society as a whole and it is a litmus test for health and social care services.' Implementation of the strategy is intended to make a step change in access to high quality care for all people approaching the end of life. The strategy makes it clear that this step change should apply irrespective of age, gender, ethnicity, religious belief, disability, sexual orientation, diagnosis, or socio-economic deprivation. The strategy also makes it clear that high quality care should be available wherever the person may be: at home, in a care home, in a hospice, or elsewhere.

The scale of the task to achieve these aims is widely recognized, but there is also wide agreement that progress can and is being made despite the constraints imposed by financial austerity.

So what contribution can *Death, Dying, and Social Differences* make to implementation of the end of life care strategy, other than reinforcing the needs of different groups? One clear message comes through to me from many of the chapters. That is the importance and value to all concerned of cross boundary working. We now have good examples of specialist palliative care teams working with dementia service providers bringing their joint expertise to the benefit of patients in their usual residence or place of care. The authors of this book have demonstrated that this approach can and should be extended by bringing together teams with expertise in the management of teenagers, people with mental health problems, or people with physical or intellectual disabilities (to give just a few examples) with those with expertise in end of life care.

Reference

Department of Health. (2008). *End of Life Care Strategy*. London: Department of Health Publications.

Index